Take Two Aspirin and Call Me at 20,000 Feet

REVIEWS AND ACCOLADES

After many years of trying to persuade my good friend and colleague, Dr. Michael Manyak, to write down his many experiences and adventures, it looks as though he has finally done it. His new book, *Take Two Aspirin and Call Me at 20,000 Feet*, does not disappoint. Mike is a former academic physician and urology department chair at George Washington University medical school where we overlapped in the 2000s. Beyond his teaching and clinical responsibilities, Dr. Manyak maintained an almost insatiable curiosity and appetite for adventure and exploration taking him to the far reaches of our planet. At the same time, Dr. Manyak never forgot his humanity and love for his fellow human beings. He always remained committed to linking his travels to helping those in need. What comes through in this book is a compelling story of both excitement and giving back – it's a terrific book.

–**Peter Hotez, MD, PhD**, Nobel Prize in Medicine nominee 2022, founding Dean US National School of Tropical Medicine

An amazing true-life story and an inspiration for others to think outside the box. Michael's life illustrates the power of following your own instincts and being prepared….a good guide for all of us.

–**Steve Elkins**, explorer, award-winning film producer, protagonist of *The Lost City of the Monkey God: A True Story* by author Douglas Preston

For those who venture to the edges of the world, Mike Manyak is the go-to source on medical matters. In this authoritative and thoroughly enjoyable memoir, we now have the insightful stories to help keep adventurers safe – and most of us alive.

–**Rick Potts**, Paleoanthropologist and Director of the Smithsonian Human Origins Program

Dr. Manyak's life is excitement with a series of surprises - like a library of the world's best novels - only it's all true and you can't predict the next scene. Mike's exceptional writing style captures the reader's interest from beginning to end. Don't expect to stop reading - once you begin. Prepare for the fireworks!

–**Rear Adm (ret) USPHS Dr. Joyce Johnson**, former Director, Health and Safety, US Coast Guard, and Fellow, The Explorers Club

Michael Manyak brings his many talents to bear as a world-class physician, explorer, and storyteller in this wonderful collection of tales from some of the world's most far-flung reaches. Laced with vivid detail and the insights of a leading expert in expedition medicine, *Take Two Aspirin and Call Me at 20,000 Feet*, weaves a page-turning narrative of adventure that takes readers from the heights of the Andes and grassy steppes of Mongolia to jungles of the Congo and the wreckage of the Titanic on the floor of the Atlantic. Dr. Manyak's new book will leave science and exploration enthusiasts hungering for more.

–**Scott Wallace**, author *The Unconquered: In Search of the Amazon's Last Uncontacted Tribes and Central America in the Crosshairs of War*. Contributing author, National Geographic Magazine.

Dr. Michael Manyak's latest book is a thrilling journey through the uncharted territories of both the world and the human spirit. With a blend of heart-pounding adventures, real-world medical dramas and occasional side-splitting humor, Dr. Manyak invites readers to join him on his fascinating life journey and his many daring escapades at the edges of a planet very few of us really know. From spine-tingling encounters on the ocean floor retrieving artifacts from the Titanic to advising NASA on aerospace medicine to laugh-out-loud pranks played by an assortment of colleagues, this book is a testament to Dr. Manyak's remarkable storytelling prowess and his unparalleled zest for life. This is an exhilarating and mind expanding read that will leave you sometimes breathless, definitely a lot wiser and occasionally in stitches. This book showcases Dr. Manyak's unique ability to turn the extraordinary into the unforgettable.

–**Warren Young**, former Director of Security, International Monetary Fund

Author and explorer Mike Manyak provides his readers with an incredible roller-coaster of emotions and excitement. While reading this book, I laughed, cried, sweated, feared, admired, worried, feared, and most of all, learned so much. This book is a masterful read of how one man not only explored the planet but also served humankind every step of the way.

—**Meg Lowman**, author *The Arbornaut*,
Farrar and awardee, The Explorers Medal 2023

Mike Manyak makes Indiana Jones look like a parochial slacker. Indeed, *Take Two Aspirin and Call me at 20,000 Feet* reads like a Hollywood action thriller; one moment the peripatetic doctor and explorer is jetting off to Morocco on a private 747 to wrangle a Saudi crown prince's anomalous kidney, the next he's abetting the extraction of semen from a rare white rhino with arthritic knees. It's a fast-paced romp through a remarkable life at the forefront of exploration and medicine, one that's as inspiring as it is hard to put down.

—**Carl Hoffman**, New York Times bestselling author
of *Savage Harvest* and *The Lunatic Express*

Spine-tingling adventure at every turn – Manyak puts you there. Turn off that reality show and live along with him!

–**Randall N. Hyer, MD, PhD, MPH**, Fellow, The Explorer's Club,
and formerly the Winter-Over Medical Officer,
Operation DEEP FREEZE, Antarctica

Like Coleridge's ancient mariner, Dr. Manyak has a tale to tell and what a collection of tales he has! The reader is taken through fascinating accounts of exploration and life adventures made even more enjoyable by Dr. Manyak's easy writing style and organization. The short chapters make it difficult to stop, and you want to read what's next on his table of delicious adventures.

–**Craig Cook, MD**, Fellow Explorers Club, Divers Alert Network (DAN),
former Medical Director Sport Dive Magazine

In *Take Two Aspirin and Call Me At 20,000 Feet*, Michael J. Manyak, MD masterfully guides readers through many of the amazing experiences he has encountered throughout his career. Mike has lived the full life that few others will ever experience, and he shares the details of his adventures in this book. Mike also provides insight into his family life and how he has been able to share some of his experiences with his children and wife. It is clear that Mike's exploits have focused on making the world a better and safer place. Mike's depth of knowledge in numerous areas is evident and his medical knowledge and ability to plan and execute detailed Crisis Management support systems is truly amazing. The world needs many more people like Mike.

–**Jeff Denton**, High Threat Security and Logistics Expert,
formerly with Triple Canopy and Constellis

TAKE TWO ASPIRIN
AND
CALL ME
AT
20,000 FEET

AN EAGLE SCOUT AT THE CROSSROADS
OF MEDICINE, EXPLORATION, & SCIENCE

Michael J. Manyak, MD

NEW YORK

LONDON • NASHVILLE • MELBOURNE • VANCOUVER

Take Two Aspirin and Call Me at 20,000 Feet

An Eagle Scout at the Crossroads of Medicine, Exploration, and Science

Published in New York, New York, by Morgan James Publishing. Morgan James is a trademark of Morgan James, LLC. www.MorganJamesPublishing.com

Proudly distributed by Publishers Group West®

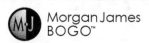

ISBN 9781636983936 paperback
ISBN 9781636984124 ebook
Library of Congress Control Number: 2023952193

Cover & Interior Design by:
Christopher Kirk
www.GFSstudio.com

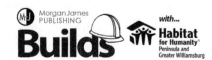

Morgan James is a proud partner of Habitat for Humanity Peninsula and Greater Williamsburg. Partners in building since 2006.

Get involved today! Visit: www.morgan-james-publishing.com/giving-back

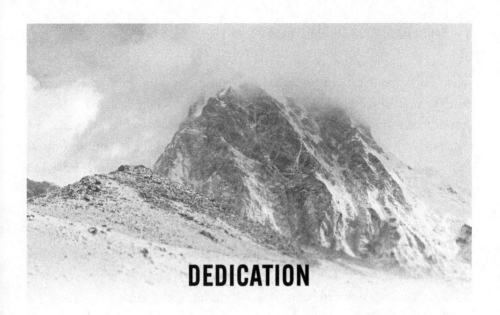

DEDICATION

This book is dedicated to different groups and individuals who have had a major influence on my life and provided significant enrichment of these stories.

First and foremost, my children Rachel, Susanna, and Timothy are the ones who cajoled and browbeat me to undertake this for they understandably cannot remember all the tales told over the years. They are most important to me. They and my wife Rebecca kept the home fires burning through all these travels and adventures. They gave me fierce reasons to return. I like to believe that I stimulated some of their curiosity for life and travel.

Close friends and colleagues with whom I have shared adventures or who have had major influences on my life and lent legitimacy to those activities include noted paleoanthropologist Rick Potts, NASA aerospace medicine expert Rich Williams, Rear Admiral (ret) Joyce Johnson, medical executive Michael Barch, infectious disease expert Peter Hotez, urologist Harry Miller, and brilliant scientists Angelo Russo and Jim Mitchell from the NCI and Steve Patierno from Duke.

High threat security friends and those from lettered agencies (CIA, NSA, DIA, FBI) have been integral to many of these stories. Scott Harrison was a frequent collaborator, closer than my relatives, instigator, agent provocateur, raconteur par excellence, and kindred spirit. Tim Weir has long believed in disease surveillance and its security implications. Bruce McIndoe is a highly experienced radiation and security expert. Triple Canopy colleagues Jeff Denton, high threat security and logistics expert, and Jay Christy, special forces helicopter pilot and noted expert marksman remain friends to this day. William Green is a senior security executive who believes in the intertwining of medical and security issues. Ric Jacobson is a road warrior security expert and friend for many years. And of course, Warren Young, is the former IMF director of security and now ex pat restaurateur and unofficial mayor of picturesque San Miguel de Allende in Mexico. What fun it would be to get that band together again.

National Eagle Scout Association executives and colleagues who have shared a dream to bring exploration to Eagle Scouts and scouts in general include Bill Steele (also a noted speleologist), Glenn Adams, Frank Tsuru, Joe Weingarten, and Rick Bragga. Our younger generation of leaders are fine in their hands.

Lastly and far from least are my explorer colleagues and friends, a fascinating group. Notable among them are anthropologist and dynamic writer Wade Davis, renowned balloonist Sir David Hempleman-Adams, arbonaut pioneer Meg Lowman, ex-fighter pilot and scuba diver Harry Brooks, dive medicine expert Craig Cook, narwhal expert Martin Nweeia, noted ornithologist Bill Bowerman, kayaker and environmental scientist Piotr Chmielinski, expedition medicine expert Ken Kamler, and astronaut Kathy Sullivan. And to those explorer friends and pioneers whom I have admired who have gone on recently to higher exploration, Ad Astra as they say at The Explorers Club: Sir Edmund Hillary, Jim Fowler, Clive Cussler, E. O. Wilson, Lee Talbot, Genie Clark, John Hare, Bill Lishman, and Don Walsh. There are many others over the years.

TABLE OF CONTENTS

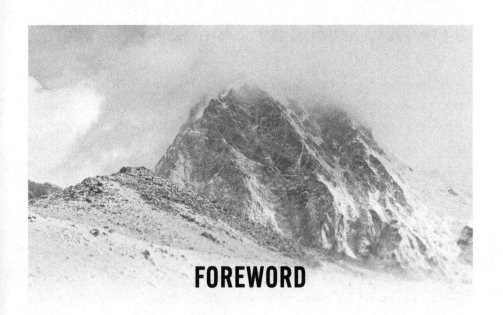

FOREWORD

"That is a tiger! Let's get closer!"
Mike Manyak, Kaziranga Game Preserve, Assam State, India 1993

By all accounts, a successful career as an academic surgeon culminating in chairmanship of a department in a major US medical university is a life-defining, pinnacle career accomplishment. For my dear friend and colleague Mike Manyak, highest academic success reflects only a single aspect of a life filled with an amazing panoply of high adventure and achievement.

I have known Mike for over 20 years. We met while I was working as NASA's Chief Health and Medical Officer. Much remains unknown about the risks attending long duration exploration class human space flight missions. We are always looking for advisors who can lend insight and experience to inform our understanding and human space flight risk mitigation strategies. Mike, a renowned explorer and expert in tropical diseases, expedition medicine, biotechnology, and urology, was a natural consultant for us. Mike and I have collaborated and remained friends since those days.

Mike's vast array of experiences are beyond remarkable. His early days as a health care first responder and his experiences with the pharmaceutical industry led him to a life in medicine. His medical education at the University of the East Ramon Magsaysay Memorial Medical Center (UERM) in Manila, Philippines, allowed him to witness and treat many tropical diseases firsthand, a rich experience resulting in world class expertise in tropical medicine. His many and varied (sometimes austere and dangerous) experiences in Manila, including a brief career in professional basketball and modeling, provided a crucible in which his many unique skills were forged.

As I read this book, I was riveted by Mike's accounts of expedition after expedition in varied disciplines all over the globe, his associations with royalty and heads of state, his forays into the world of international security services (including medical services for combatants worldwide), his leadership activities in the Explorers Club, his contributions to the National Eagle Scout Association and so much more. Mike discusses a genetic variant thought to drive the human exploration imperative – if such a variant exists, it reaches highest expression in Mike Manyak.

I chose Mike's tiger quote as the theme of this endorsement because it epitomizes his approach to life. With high adventure comes high risk; you can't do the things Mike has done without embracing, understanding, accepting, and effectively managing those risks. Throughout an amazing career and life, Mike Manyak has come very close to the tiger indeed. I'm sure you will enjoy reading about it as much as I have.

–**Richard Williams** MD MPH FACS, Col, USAF (ret)
Former NASA Chief Health and Medical Officer
Former Health Director, Virginia Department of Health

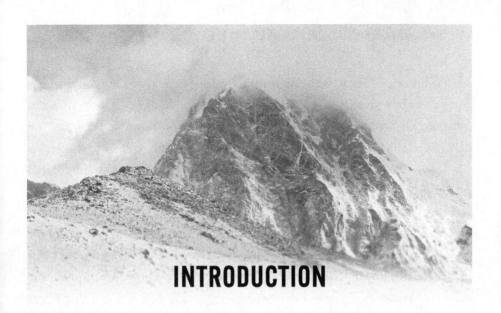

INTRODUCTION

Have you excavated early human artifacts in Africa? Operated a submersible at the Titanic wreck site? Been on foot up close with the newly described, highly endangered, third species of camel deep in the Gobi Desert?

Have you had to intubate the trachea of a gorilla to give it anesthesia? Have you operated on rhinos, a very rare cat species, gorillas, or a huge boar hog? Have you been charged by an enraged lion or a trumpeting furious elephant? Not faux charges. Been on foot up close with rhinos?

What about finding sunken Spanish treasure? Been caught in a coup in a dangerous third-world country? Witnessed the Pentagon attack on 9/11? Evacuated an injured patient from deep in the Andes? Have you been personally involved in healthcare of foreign and national heads of state? Managed exotic venomous snake bites and evacuation? Learned how to drive out of an ambush that killed the driver while you were riding shotgun? Waltzed through the Berlin Zoo at midnight smoking a cigar? Rescued nearly one hundred victims from a sinking ship?

Although seemingly disconnected, the common threads of medicine and exploration are intertwined in these events. Combining medicine with adventure has been the dominant theme in my life. At times I have been afforded a ringside seat for historical events, while on occasion, I have been thrust into unusual circumstances by chance. I have shaken my head in wonderment on more than one occasion. My life has never been boring. My guiding principle has been that you may not be able to make life longer, but you CAN make it wider.

I have worn several hats throughout life and the reader will gain insight into the thought processes of becoming an academic cancer surgeon who lends his expertise to exploration both in the field sciences and in the lab. This book has clinical experiences in urology and tropical medicine interspersed with remote expeditions very much as they happened. Along the way you will meet quite a cast of characters, some of them household names and others better left in the dusty corners of history.

Buckle your chinstrap and come on board.

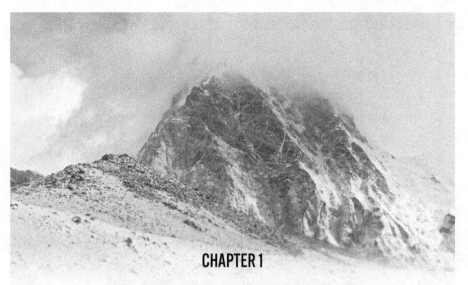

CHAPTER 1

SOUTH CHINA SEA RESCUE

The commotion on deck penetrated my rum-aided sleep at 3:00 a.m. The crew of our dive boat were fishing a woman from the turbulent sea five miles from shore. She had been clinging to wooden debris in the choppy rolling waves seemingly alone in the ocean. Between sobs she told us that more than 100 people had been dumped into the sea from an overloaded inter-island vessel that had capsized eight hours earlier. The vessel, typical in the Philippines, had also been transporting chickens, pigs, bags of rice and many passengers beyond its capacity. A Russian oil tanker had drawn close to the vessel, its large wake panicked the passengers who ran to the opposite side, causing the ship to capsize. The woman was crying that she had lost two sons in the accident. We quickly realized there must be other victims in the ocean.

The women divers on board immediately started making coffee, getting drinks and towels and t-shirts to share with the accident victims. The men scrambled to focus strong lights on the ocean where faint cries sounded like ghosts from the unseen victims in the five-foot chop. Consistent with the poor safety standards of these types of vessels, the few lifeboats that were launched were dysfunctional and overloaded. This became evident when we came upon one of them partially sunken with eighteen people, mostly children, crammed into it, water up to their chests.

It was heartbreaking to see that the three adults were passing around an eight-month-old baby and had been rotating from person to person. This had been going on for eight hours. The other older children hung precariously onto thin ropes as the waves washed over them. Over the course of seven hours, we pulled in eighty-seven people, many of them children, onto our 75-foot dive boat.

This rescue was like a religious experience. These people would have been dead had we not run across them. Fortunately, the turbulence in the water distracted any sharks from finding them yet but it was only a matter of time. As a newly minted medical school graduate and the only doctor on board, the medical responsibilities fell on me. Fortunately, we only had a few people who required medical attention, one with a significant laceration and a few others who had swallowed too much seawater.

My extensive ambulance experience and Eagle Scout training had partially prepared me for this type of experience when there were available resources. However, in this remote area, with no obvious resources except a first aid kit, we were pretty much on our own. The situation was tragic and highly emotional; there were still many people hanging on for dear life out in the ocean. We attempted to contact the U.S. Naval Air Base at Subic Bay although it was not clear that our message was received. However, we were able to signal a passing fishing vessel and later learned from newspaper reports that the fishermen rescued about the same number of people we did. This meant that the actual toll from this disaster was significantly less than expected.

We proceeded on to the Negros Occidental provincial capital of Mamburao with the victims to a small hospital. On the way into Mamburao, we came across a viable lifeboat, surprising since the ones we had come across were damaged. We learned that the captain and purser were on this lifeboat; apparently, they had abandoned ship and the passengers in the water, absconding with the money on the boat. The silence of the passengers and the ship's crew created an ominous atmosphere. As they neared our boat, one of them cut the line and they drifted off. I was told that the passengers might have killed the captain and crew for abandoning them and taking one of the only functioning lifeboats. Maritime justice indeed.

After several hours of rescue work, a small group of us went ashore after daybreak and banged on the door of the local hospital. A doctor answered sleepily and realized he faced his worst nightmare. Fortunately, the people we rescued weren't badly hurt and we left them, having been assured they would get proper care.

This traumatic situation prompted me to reflect about what you must do in remote situations with few resources if trouble occurs. Saving these lives emphasized that personal and group safety were extremely important in austere environments. This experience inspired me to get involved with what became my life's passion – expedition medicine.

Meanwhile, after replenishing our stores as best we could, we proceeded to our destination, Apo Reef, near the island of Palawan famous for its crystal-clear waters and a reef wall that goes beyond forty meters. This premier spot for scuba diving is an archipelagic province in the westernmost region in the Philippines located 490 miles southwest of Manila. The voyage there was beautiful with flying fish landing on board and dolphins accompanying us against a backdrop of a spectacular sunset. We arrived at night and promptly embarked on a night dive.

Night dives require different safety parameters because your only visibility is provided by hand-carried lights. If your light goes out or is lost, it is pitch black and you may not know which way is up to the surface. It is very important to use the buddy system on this type of dive and bubbles, though not well seen, always rise so you know which way to go.

It is rather disconcerting if you are not used to night diving, but the dives are breathtaking. The extremely colorful coral polyps, reminiscent of circus clown flowers, are not visible in daytime but now extend into the water. Goliath groupers, the size of large tables, are asleep and you can approach them and tap on their sides without them moving. If you shut off your lights and wave your arms, the phosphorescent plankton lights up like Christmas lights. It is spectacularly beautiful. Such was our second night on this dive trip.

This was the maiden voyage for the dive boat, and our hostess and owner of the dive boat, Maryanne (Ma'an) Hontiveros, was a celebrity in the Philippines who produced and starred in a weekly news magazine show. Our group of about twenty-five included very experienced divers, even a couple of the top spearfisher-men in the islands. Close friend Scott Harrison, frequent co-conspirator in mis-chief and accomplished scuba diver who spurred my diving interest, was aboard; later he would be the CIA station chief in several countries. Ma'an had her film crew record the sea rescue and dive highlights. After the sea disaster and rescue, she intended to have an expose' decrying the flagrant disregard of safety issues and the over manifest of passengers and cargo. Unfortunately, most of the film was ruined in Manila while being processed.

For me, the 1979 sea rescue experience both illuminated and cemented my interest in remote medical care and expedition and wilderness medicine. I thought I was on an adventure celebrating the end of my medical school educa-tion. Instead, I was ushering in the beginning of something significant in my life. From this point on, I was determined to seek opportunities to collaborate with major national and international organizations in global travel. My contribution would be medical preparation and safety. Medicine was my career and urology my chosen discipline. Expedition and wilderness medicine was now my avocation.

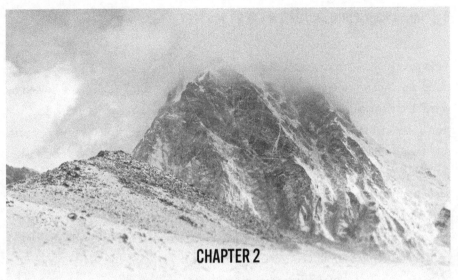

CHAPTER 2

DOWN TO THE TITANIC

T houghts about that rescue would crop up on occasion. As I became more known among explorers for my medical expertise, I was contacted in early 2000 by a close Explorers Club friend, Dave Concannon, a maritime law attorney who had helped negotiate the agreement between the State of Florida and the discoverers of the *Senora Nuestra de Atocha*, the most famous Spanish treasure galleon found. This time he was calling me to see if I could provide medical services for the upcoming *RMS Titanic* salvage operation. This was a proposed six-week expedition in the North Atlantic and would involve fifty Americans and about seventy-five Russian crew and scientists who operated the research vessel that housed the submersibles.

I am often asked to name my favorite expedition and my usual answer is "the next one," but it is hard to top this unique experience. My responsibility as the medical officer was to provide expertise, supplies, medical evacuation insurance, and personnel for the expedition. The plan was to deploy the MIR submersibles from the Russian oceanic research vessel *Akademik Mstislav Keldysh* to search for artifacts. These were the same submersibles used in the movie Titanic with the same captain and sub pilots. The *AM Keldysh* is a 6240-ton 7 deck vessel owned by the Shirsov Institute of Oceanology of the Russian Academy of Sciences. The fifty non-Russian members ranged from scientists and explorers to investors, actors, and even an out-of-work rock band. It was quite a motley crew to say the least.

Although a few high-priced tourist trips have visited the site, this was the second official dive to retrieve artifacts. RMS Titanic, Inc., the privately held company, held the salvage rights to the *Titanic*. The right to salvage involves "arresting" the ship in question which requires an artifact retrieved from the site that is registered in an admiralty court. In this case, this was done by this company in a Virginia admiralty court. Even though the *Titanic* originated from Great Britain and was designated a Royal Mail Ship (hence the RMS prefix), salvage rights were awarded to a U.S.-based company.

The *Titanic* site is near the fishing grounds of Grand Banks, the site of the wreck of the *Andrea Gail* depicted in the movie "The Perfect Storm" which was released the previous year. Hurricanes are relatively rare in that area, but many people not involved expressed concern about another such storm which I scoffed at. As I waited in the quaint city of St. John's in Newfoundland to take my two-week turn at sea, we watched a tropical storm in the Caribbean roll up the US East Coast, waiting for it to make landfall. To the delight of the meteorologists and to my horror, it avoided land and headed right out to the North Atlantic. The seas are notoriously rough even on good days in that location with a swell that can be ten to fifteen feet, making transfer and resupply from the smaller vessels onto the large Russian research vessel *Keldysh* quite treacherous. A hurricane was not welcome news.

We had no word about the research ships for three days, but the *Keldysh* finally signaled its return to the site after going 250 miles to avoid the storm. After three successive nights of bon voyage parties with too much of the local nasty rum, it was time to get out to sea if nothing more than to save our livers. It was only after debriefing my medical colleague, also an Army Ranger instructor used to crisis, who went on the first two-week leg of the expedition that we learned how close the other smaller research vessel came to sinking. His stateroom was "upside down" and he had the now terrified scientists and crew put on life preservers and be prepared to go in the water. Fortunately, the captain came to his senses and evacuated.

This was only one of the unusual events during this expedition. We only had five days to dive into the *Titanic* site with the two submersibles because that hurricane made an about-face and came roaring back, so we had to leave. We weathered other problems as well. Five patients had medical problems, three of them with painful kidney stones, though none were obstructing the urinary tract which would necessitate a complicated emergency evacuation. A fourth female patient had a complex ovarian cystic mass suggestive of cancer which we diagnosed with the ultrasound (as we did the urinary stones) we brought. Funny how all the jokes ceased about why we had a urologist and gynecologist as doctors on this trip. They had better subspecialty care than at home. The site was thirty-six hours from the nearest port making a water-borne evacuation impractical. Helicopters could not land on the *Keldysh* because of limited landing space and overhead wires leaving the only route for evacuation an off-board basket rescue after a tricky midair refueling operation.

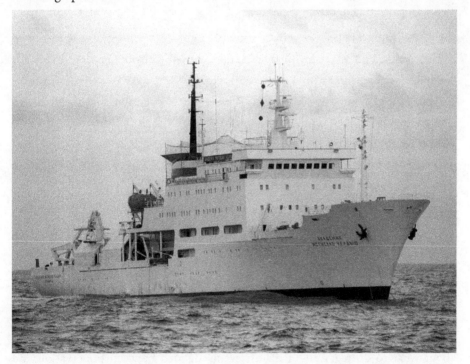

The *Akademik Keldysh* Russian marine research vessel from which MIR submersibles were deployed.

Therefore, it was advisable to deal with medical emergencies on site if possible. Fortunately, the Russians had a small surgical suite that could be used for basic procedures. Even something straightforward like an appendectomy could be challenging if there were complications or anatomical variations like a retrocecal appendix. Compounding this was the problem of anesthesia. The Russians had ether, a standard anesthetic forty years earlier but now rarely used as an anesthetic agent because of its volatility and flammability.

The Russians who ran the program and research ship were consummate professionals and, fortunately, there were some qualified individuals among the fifty expedition members. Some of the remainder of the crew concealed serious medical conditions, jeopardizing their safety and the overall mission.

This is precisely what you worry about as a medical officer. Expedition members are prone to hide medical conditions if they think they will be scrubbed from the mission, not realizing (or ignoring) that if they become ill it is not only their health that may be compromised but that of the entire mission. For example, at sea, I was approached by one of the sound engineers working on the film who disclosed that he had major prostate surgery three weeks before departure, still had a urinary catheter in place, and was leaking urine.

He should never have been on the trip, not to mention that the Russians wanted to dismember him for leaking in their submersible. In other circumstances, the medical officer may have to accompany a sick or injured patient to more sophisticated care. This delays the expedition and may leave the expedition without an experienced medical person in a potentially dangerous situation.

Other unanticipated problems faced were not easily bypassed. A crew member attempted suicide and had to be evacuated, leaving a gap in the command structure at the top. This issue arose because the leader of the expedition and president of RMS Titanic, Inc., had learned right after we arrived on the *Keldysh* that in his absence, the other three members of their board had called an emergency meeting, appointed a fifth member to the board by a split vote, and then voted to remove him from the board and as president. The board had been deadlocked about what to do regarding artifacts, evenly divided between preservation and public exhibition versus selling the artifacts on eBay. This expedition was the culmination of years of effort and cost by the president, and he was adamant about not selling artifacts. So, the opposing side decided to remove him. Furthermore, they informed him that his wife, the corporate attorney, had misbehaved while on shore waiting for the hurricane to pass.

You can imagine the dual impact of their call. He was very agitated shortly after I arrived on board, but I did not know the cause. He then said he had to return to shore to sort out this mess and he left on the zodiac at night. Halfway across the 400-meter gap between the *Keldysh* and our supply boat which we had arrived on, he stood up in the zodiac, turned to the small crew, and declared it was a great night for a swim and jumped overboard without a life preserver.

Fortunately, the two Irish Marine divers with him jumped in and wrestled him back into the zodiac. He proceeded on back to Canada and we were left without the expedition leader. By default, the director of security, a former British SAS major, became the expedition leader. Although I got along well with him, some other members of the crew objected to his method of discipline and there was palpable dissension. As is common in such circumstances, many turned to the doctor to be the peacemaker. I was in the middle of this controversy despite my protests and there was an uneasy truce for the remainder of the trip. None of this involved the Russians who were the consummate professionals, completing the dives according to schedule and objectives.

The cook was not sober the entire time, terrifying me that he would start a fire in the galley, cut off his finger, or create an epidemic of bacterial diarrhea. We joked about checking the salad for extra condiments. Also, on the return to Canada with the artifacts, the engines suddenly stopped, and we learned that the Russians had not been paid so we were hostages in international waters without legal jurisdiction until that was corrected. There were some tense moments indeed. We certainly welcomed the sight of the Newfoundland signal tower which received the SOS from the *Titanic* on that fateful day in 1912 that now indicated we were back home.

A very poignant event occurred shortly after I arrived on the *Keldysh*. The director of the submersible program came to me with an urgent and confidential matter to discuss. Dr. Anatoly Sagalevich is a Russian explorer who developed the submersibles which were ingeniously modified Soyuz space capsules. Anatoly holds the record for the deepest freshwater dive in Lake Baikal and after multiple

Titanic dives, he later went on expeditions to the German battleship *Bismarck* and both Soviet and Japanese sunken submarines.

Anatoly explained he had received an urgent request from the Russian government and President Putin personally to aid in a national emergency. The Russian nuclear submarine *Kursk* had sustained an accident and could not surface, trapping several sailors. It was unknown how many of the 118 personnel were still alive. Unfortunately, we were in the North Atlantic, far from the site of the disaster in the Sea of Murmansk. All of us on the *Keldysh* were very somber and commiserated with our Russian colleagues. Anatoly explained that I might be needed as a doctor if we could get to the submarine. Unfortunately, we could not get there in time even if we left immediately and we could only await updates on the sailors' fate. There were no survivors.

As a follow up to the *Kursk* story, about two weeks after I had returned to clinical duties at GW, I had a U.S. Naval intelligence officer patient in for a routine visit. I told him my story of being on call to help the *Kursk*. He then told me the cause of the *Kursk* accident was a malfunction of a torpedo which exploded in the sub, killing several instantly but also trapping twenty-three sailors in a forward hold where they survived for over six hours. The initial explosion caused other torpedoes to explode. The Russians had disabled the emergency rescue buoy, so no one knew about the disaster for more than six hours. What a tragedy.

What was it like to be on the ocean floor 2.5 miles below the surface collecting artifacts from the historic wreck? The salvage expedition to the *Titanic* was intended to have a dive by each of the MIR Submersibles daily for three weeks. Unfortunately, the hurricane made an about face and headed back towards us, so we had to cut short the excursion. The hurricane in the area significantly limited dives to a total of ten from the two submersibles so I was extremely fortunate to have been on one of them. More people have flown in space than have gone to the Titanic.

The pre-dive briefing with the MIR pilots reviewed responsibilities of the three-man crew and objectives of our twelve-hour mission. The most experienced Russian sub pilot was at the helm for my descent, and I was selected as co-pilot with duties to help log and videotape each artifact in three dimensions at discovery and submit them for identification and preservation to the curator and chief marine archaeologist aboard the mother ship research vessel.

The submersibles are engineering marvels, reconfigured Russian Soyuz space capsules with three 8-inch -thick acrylic portholes to peer through the sub's 1.5-inch reinforced titanium hull. The retractable, facile robotic arms could move in any direction and retrieve either heavy pieces or very delicate artifacts.

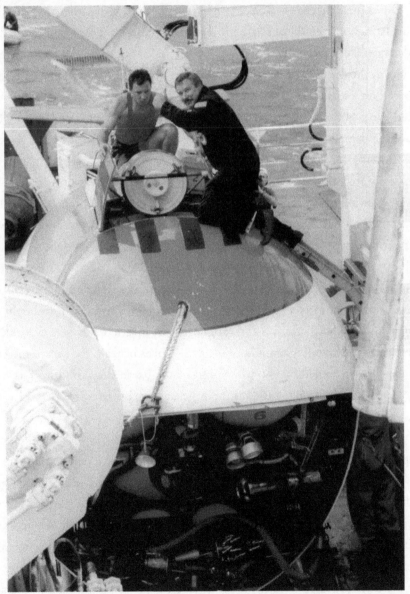

Entering Russian Mir submersible reconfigured from Soyuz space capsule

Sub deployment requires extensive coordination to guide it from its protective berth on deck into the water. Once in the turbulent water, a crewmember had to jump onto the sub, disconnect the heavy top cable and attach a smaller one to its nose, then tow it 500 meters before descent.

During the short tow from the *Keldysh*, the pilot tested the controls while a Russian sailor rode the sub like a water skier and then jumped off as we dove underwater. For nearly three hours we slowly spiraled down at a rate of 25 meters a minute to the ocean floor nearly 2.5 miles from the surface. Light sources, oxygen and carbon dioxide levels, communications, and other critical functions were tested every 500 meters. Inside the cramped cabin, the temperature started at a steamy 85 degrees but dropped nearly 40 degrees by the time we hit ocean bottom.

Visibility was quite good for the first 150 meters, though we saw no aquatic life. The water was opaque below a few hundred feet but was surprisingly clear when we switched on the lights. From that point throughout our slow, twirling descent we saw an amazing spectrum of marine life. What looked like silt were masses of tiny unidentified creatures paddling frantically while bright red shrimp and intricate jellyfish, one with a bright red internal globe like a Christmas ornament, cruised by the sub. This regatta was quite unexpected. Large rattail fish proved quite inquisitive. Several lobster species ranged in color from bright red to opalescent. Ghostly starfish and various marine invertebrates were everywhere. There was an astounding amount of life at 2.5 miles beneath the ocean surface.

Finally, we landed on the white sand of the ocean floor 1000 meters from the wreck. As we navigated toward the wreckage, we began to see large pieces of *Titanic* debris.

And then suddenly, there it was! The gigantic ghostly bow of the 883-foot-long *Titanic* was more awesome than I imagined and looked just like the famous photos. Slowly, we cruised along the bow, passing Captain James Smith's berth with his porcelain bathtub still intact, open to view because of the crease from the iceberg. Damage from the iceberg was still apparent on the hull. We inspected the large rift where the rupture separated the stern from the bow that was well depicted in the movie.

We then glided on to the large debris field that surrounds the stern, separated 600 meters from the bow. The ocean floor here is littered with evidence of the tragedy which spilled from the sinking ship: dishes with the White Star Line logo, pieces of furniture, personal items, chandeliers, portholes, candelabra.

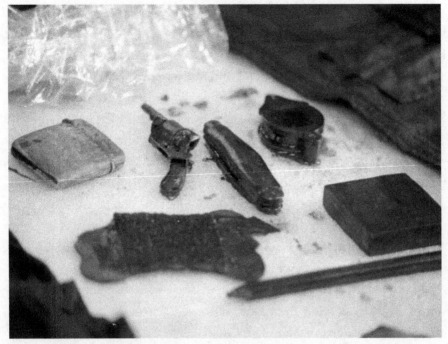

Artifacts from the *Titanic* including a flint case of non-surviving third-class passenger William Henry Allen.
Toy pistol for his son and preserved omnibus ticket which brought him to the ship

The occasional suitcase was a treasure trove because the tanning process of the leather preserved many otherwise perishable items. The organisms that usually metabolize cloth, paper and other perishables do not like the chemicals used in the tanning process. One suitcase contained the suits, shoes, jeweler's loop, pen-knife, and other personal items of William Allen III, who did not survive the trip. It was very poignant to see his engraved lighter, his completely intact and readable London omnibus tickets in his pocket, and the toy pistol gift for his son.

We came upon a man's derby on the ocean floor, still intact after all these years, and retrieved it with the robotic arm. A large cannister turned out to be a tea service for this British ship. One of the most significant artifacts we retrieved was the telegraph that connected the engine room to the bridge. Its lever would have been pushed to change course and speed when the iceberg was sighted. Nowhere were there any human remains; at 6000 pounds per square inch of pressure in slightly acidic water due to the calcium carbonate, those remains were long since pulverized and dissolved.

My greatest thrill occurred when the sub pilot allowed me the rarely afforded honor to pilot the submersible on the ocean floor and use the robotic arms to retrieve artifacts. Using the dual control joysticks, this fascinating tactile experience was remarkably like laparoscopic and robotic surgery that I had performed which is the reason he allowed me to do this.

Before ascent the sub pilot produced a picnic basket replete with sandwiches and a good champagne, both of which we consumed with gusto. After six hours on the ocean floor, we reluctantly began the process of ascent. I had been totally immersed in the dive experience, but now certain needs have reasserted themselves. Portable urinals are available on the sub, but the pilots never seem to use them. Later, I discovered the reason: they have a standing bet whereby the first pilot who succumbs to the temptation must contribute a bottle of scotch to be consumed by the others once topside.

Nearly three hours after beginning our ascent we were gratified to hear the voice from the bridge of the *Keldysh* signaling that we were near the surface. After surfacing, the MIR bobbed in the swells of the North Atlantic and I thought this must be how the astronauts felt as they awaited recovery in their space capsule after splashdown. Soon we were towed back to the mother ship and hoisted on deck and the artifacts submitted to the curator for preservation. We were giddy with exhilaration as we clambered out the hatch to the cheers of the crew.

Among the 853 artifacts recovered during the expedition were the captain's wheel, which Captain Smith is said to have held onto while going down with the ship, the base of the cherub statue from the grand

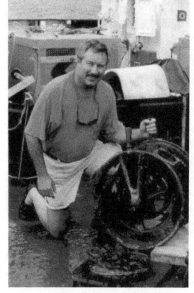

The telegraph that connected the bridge and the engine room when the iceberg was sighted that sank the *Titanic*.

staircase and the watertight seal of the door that, had it been closed, would have prevented the ship from sinking before the *Carpathia* came to the rescue.

The magnitude of what we had been able to do left a residual glow that lingered for weeks after we returned. Now, when I think back, some of the exhilaration returns. I remain grateful for such a fantastic experience which remains vivid to this day.

But I was not done with the *Titanic*. There have been occasional returns to the *Titanic* site by wealthy tourists who paid steep sums to view the wreck. Some of these were on the Russian MIR submersibles but others were with private company vehicles with questionable safety parameters.

The world was transfixed when the carbon fiber-hulled OceanGate submersible *Titan* disappeared about two hours after it had submerged June 18, 2023. When the media asked for my opinion, I said that when they had not resurfaced a few hours after they lost communication, it likely signified a catastrophic event. An intelligence expert told me at the time that the U.S. Navy would know what happened. Sure enough, the Navy had detected an acoustic signature consistent with an implosion. This meant an instantaneous death for the five passengers. A few days later, a debris field consistent with such an event was located. The submersible had not been certified below 4000 feet and carbon fiber is known to be unstable. Final analysis of the recovered artifacts has not been completed at the time of this writing.

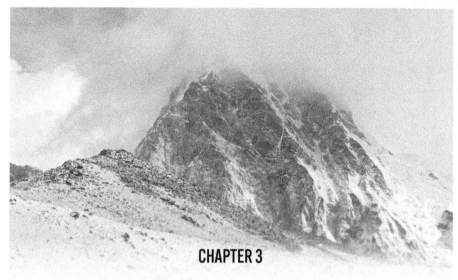

CHAPTER 3

A SURGEON'S MENTALITY

I am often asked how I became involved in expedition medicine and able to go on fantastic expeditions. The common thread is medicine because every expedition must consider safety and health aspects particularly in remote locations. While explorers may have a specific geographical area of concentration, expedition medicine encompasses all climates and geographies. There are certain common problems encountered on any expedition like transportation, the need for evacuation, and trauma while there are also concerns specific to the location that must be addressed. You can imagine that an expedition to the desert has different issues than one to high altitude or the jungle.

It all started with my medical training. I am a urologist which is a surgical specialist. Instead of doing surgical procedures in all areas of the body, my area of concentration is the urinary tract and male genital tract. There are many jokes about why someone chooses urology and I think I have heard them all over the course of my career and at cocktail parties. The succinct response I like the best is that pee is the easiest body substance to wash off your hands. That usually elicits a laugh but if it doesn't, you are probably in the wrong conversation.

Urology is an appealing field of study because you combine taking care of most medical problems related to the urinary tract such as urinary tract infections, urinary stone management, urinary obstruction in males in its initial stages (females rarely have urinary obstruction), male infertility, urinary incontinence, and male sexual dysfunction. On the other end of the spectrum are the problems that must be tackled with surgery including mechanical relief of urinary obstruction, kidney and bladder stone removal, reconstructive surgery for congenital or acquired anomalies, and some of the most common types of cancer in humans (prostate, bladder, kidney, and more rarely testicular and genital tumors). This must be done with compassion and awareness that we are dealing with one of the most emotionally and physically sensitive, and intensely private areas of the body. A urologist also often becomes the de facto primary care physician for men, much like the role gynecologists perform for women. Urologists must understand other diseases and their impact on urological or sexual function, renew common prescriptions, and refer patients to the appropriate specialty if needed.

How do you become a urologist? It takes four years of medical school and then five or six years (depending on the program) of additional training and experience in urology. When I trained, two years of general surgery was required before the next four years of urology. During those two years you learn much about patient management both before and after surgery and how to deal surgically with other organs, such as the bowel, that you will encounter in your urological surgery career. Once your six years of training is completed, you must pass your boards, an intense two-part series of written and oral exams, before you are board certified, a desirable designation. You can practice if training is complete without board certification, but most hospitals now require such status. Other training graduates can elect to go on to further specialization in a fellowship program. My fellowship was at the National Cancer Institute in an area called experimental phototherapy, an esoteric field in which one becomes an expert in lasers and special applications of laser technology.

As a urologic surgeon, you are the master and commander of the operating room for procedures. In big cases, this often involves orchestration of thirty or forty various auxiliary personnel of doctors, nurses, and technicians who are helping manage the patient physiologically or assisting directly with the surgery. The key person with whom you work with is the anesthesiologist who must have the patient in a physiologically suspended state deep enough not to feel pain or move but also able to be resuscitated to normal function. As a surgeon, you must be focused, calm, and decisive. There is a great deal of cooperation and communication needed during a surgical case and you are the maestro of this orchestra.

A perfect example of this coordination is the uncommon case referred to me from another medical center. The patient was a seventy-six-year rather frail woman who had a huge kidney tumor with growth extending from the kidney into the renal vein and up the vena cava into the right side of the heart. The surgeon had to remove the large bulky tumor, a difficult process alone, but also remove this tumor extension going into the heart. Since this involved going into the chest as well as the abdomen, I asked our experienced cardiothoracic surgeon to assist me. These tumor extensions could grow into the vena cava wall necessitating a more involved procedure with a large vein graft but more often they were slightly adherent without invading the vascular wall and could be peeled off and removed. One major concern is that if a part of the tumor extension is dislodged, the patient can have a fatal stroke.

Because of the location and size of the tumor extension and attached clot, the patient was put on cardiopulmonary bypass which mechanically takes over the circulatory function of the heart while surgical removal occurs. It is an artificial heart outside of the body. The kidney receives 20 percent of your blood volume each minute, thus the risk of extensive bleeding is always present with kidney surgery. In this case, we had to mobilize the kidney with a large bulky tumor and control the aberrant vessels. Then the vena cava, a very large vessel the size of a garden hose, was opened and the tumor carefully extracted from up in the heart. This process involved a great deal of coordination with approximately thirty people in the operating room. The cardiovascular surgeon and I ran the show. We had discussed our roles beforehand including management of any complications that arose. It was exhilarating to complete this case successfully. The patient lived another five years without any tumor recurrence and died of other causes.

All this training and development of mind set molds your personality. You become better at filtering insignificant items from the task at hand. You learn discipline, both mental and physical. You develop compassion and acceptance that all things do not work out perfectly despite intricate advance planning. You learn that your personality may not mesh with some other types. You do not suffer fools easily. Patience may be difficult. These are your shortcomings. It is important to recognize these issues. And to understand that you can learn and improve.

You must know the limits of your abilities. That is the key to being a good surgeon - know thy limitations. Do not tackle that complex problem or huge tumor if it is beyond your capabilities. Some of the most difficult cases I have had involved other urologists and other surgeons who have gotten in over their heads and needed to call for the cavalry as an emergency. We have all gotten into difficulties when you need another experienced pair of hands and eyes. If you are anticipating a potential problem that may require a different surgical specialist, it is best to plan to schedule that person to join you.

Surgery can be very intense when you are treating a difficult problem. There are some key principles you must remember. One is to operate from a known area to the unknown. This is relevant in large, complicated tumors which may be plastered on blood vessels that can lead to disaster if you cut without control of them. If you have a good outcome, it's better to stop before causing harm. Picture wanting to take a little bit more tissue, one more nibble, and then suddenly you cut into a blood vessel, or you have sheared off a delicate piece of tissue important for the repair.

A critical principle I learned from the chief of surgery, a wise experienced doctor, who always said you cannot think and yell at the same time, so you better take a deep breath instead of throwing instruments. This is so true in times of trouble, like when you inadvertently poke a hole in the aorta. Put a finger or surgical sponge on the hole, assess and catch your breath, and think about the instruments you need to fix this problem, and plan your next step. Once you release the sponge or your finger, you better be ready to move because the patient could bleed out in a minute.

It is amazing how often the principles learned in surgery come into play in settings outside the operating room. Several times I have run across bad accidents and had to jump in as a passerby Good Samaritan to stabilize significantly injured victims. I have had to evacuate injured people on remote expeditions and the reaction from my training has been the same. Everything slows down and you are laser focused. This very same phenomenon has happened to me in difficult surgical cases in times of trouble. This degree of concentration is difficult to explain, and you cannot summon it at will. It just happens and later you wonder at this phenomenon. I do not know if it is a gift or product of training but is probably a little bit of both.

An example of this occurred when I was attending a wedding in Pennsylvania shortly after my training; there was a very bad accident at the front of the country club, the site of the rehearsal dinner. We wondered why traffic was stopped and when I got out to investigate, I saw a pickup truck that had been t-boned by a Cadillac. The police had just arrived, and I went to offer my services. The Cadillac had pulled out and slammed into the pickup and the truck driver was badly injured with probable pelvic and lower back fractures. I had to focus and run through trauma protocols while people were yelling and running around. We stabilized him and awaited the ambulance to properly move him with minimal displacement of the spinal column. I then went to see who was injured in the Cadillac and found the older driver and his middle-aged daughter. Both were significantly inebriated, and the woman was screaming at me to save her father. He was not in as bad a shape and the daughter was not injured. Guardian angels watch over drunks and little kids.

The first thing one must do in emergency situations is control the crowd and take charge of the site. In this case the police were there already, a good thing since a large crowd including many of the wedding attendees had now gathered. This wedding was for a classmate of mine from Notre Dame, so I had several friends there. I was able to mobilize a couple of hulking Notre Dame football linebacker buddies to help move the patient from the truck. Others kept everyone back and out of the way of the extraction. Fortunately, no one was trapped in either vehicle.

Once everyone was sent to the hospital, I turned to the police and offered my credentials and business card. They thanked me profusely and then looked at the loud daughter who was yelling and they said, "Doc, don't worry, we never saw you," meaning that the information would not be given to the obnoxious drunk daughter. I think she was going to be sleeping someplace other than the hospital, possibly the local jail. Most of the time we do this type of work with a few witnesses and then move on.

Several times I have responded to the request from flight attendants for a doctor. In my experience, I have often had psychiatrists or pediatricians as the co-responders. With all due respect to their expertise, rarely do they have experience with emergency responses. So, you must respectfully take charge just like you would at an accident scene. Usually after getting some medical history from either the patient or a companion, you can get an idea of the problem which fortunately is often minor in nature.

Sometimes unexpected emergencies can be more serious. One time on the two-hour flight to Bermuda, I responded to find a passenger seated in the back of the plane by the flight attendants. He was overweight, pale, sweating profusely, and had some shortness of breath. He had chest pain radiating down his left arm. Although he had no history of heart problems, this was the classic presentation of an acute myocardial infarction, a heart attack.

I told the anxious family that he would be all right but needed to get to the hospital when we landed. We placed him flat on the ground with a blanket and I told the flight attendants to keep everyone out of this area. I further instructed them to notify the captain that we needed an ambulance waiting for us on the tarmac. Since we were essentially equidistant from North Carolina and Bermuda, about an hour either way, the pilot elected to continue to Bermuda which was fine. I was familiar with the medical facilities in Bermuda which would be sufficient for this problem.

There is not much you can do about this type of problem on a plane. There was a defibrillator to shock the heart if he arrested but not much else, just a nasal cannula for oxygen from a small portable tank. Running an arrest on the plane would likely be impossible. I told the flight attendants to ask for aspirin from the passengers. A myocardial infarct usually involves a blood clot in one or more cardiac vessels and an aspirin would interfere with platelet function that forms the clot. This may prevent propagation of the clot and further cardiac damage until the patient could be evaluated properly in a medical setting and possibly receive medication directly infused into his vessels to break up a clot.

The flight attendant came rushing back with an aspirin which I had the patient take with a sip of water, all the time reassuring him he would be fine, and trying to calm him, which is one of the key components for acute care in this type of situation. He did not get worse as we landed in Bermuda; we got him off to the waiting ambulance and I told the EMTs what I had done and my opinion of his condition. The man still had chest pain, but it had diminished. I gave the patient my card and best wishes and provided my information to the flight attendants.

Afterwards, American Airlines contacted me and gave me two business class seats for travel and thanked me for my assistance. I wondered what happened to the patient but did not receive any feedback. Then three months later, I received a letter from the patient with big letters THANK YOU! THANK YOU! THANK YOU! He went on to explain he had sustained a massive myocardial infarction, and the ER staff and cardiology team told him I saved his life by giving the aspirin in the middle of the event. We got him through it! There is no better feeling.

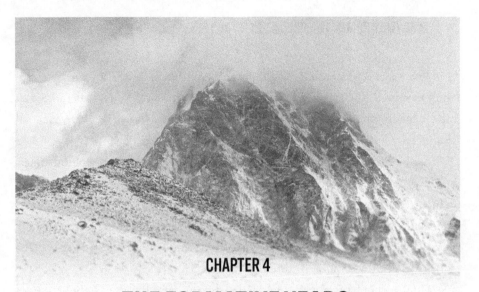

CHAPTER 4

THE FORMATIVE YEARS: DINOSAURS TO THE GOLDEN DOME

My interest in the sciences leading to medicine started at an early age. I decided at age five that I was going to be a paleontologist and hunt for dinosaur fossils. My mother got me a set of small plastic dinosaurs which I staged among the plants in our yard as I memorized their names. This was when not much was known about dinosaurs among our school-aged peers. Word got around about my unusual interest and a year later while in first grade, I was asked to share my knowledge about dinosaurs with a lecture to the 11th and 12th-grade biology classes.

My parents told me that several of their friends who had children in those classes were impressed with my presentation. My interests expanded over the years to other extinct fauna going back to the Devonian Period and into the age of mammals. Likewise, I took a strong interest in archaeology and paleoanthropology. Clearly, I was headed to a career in field science.

Flint was a mid-sized city in the lower peninsula of Michigan with a population of about 200,000 people at the time. Unfortunately, now it is more well known for its problems with a polluted water supply, but it is where General Motors (GM) was founded.

Many of the inhabitants, known affectionately by the locals as Flintstones, were involved with the automobile industry, whether it was working in a factory or involved with parts and supplies. We were no exception: my father was an engineer in the offices of AC Spark Plug, a division of GM. Times were generally prosperous during my youth and only took a downturn in the mid to late 1970s coincident to the declining fortunes of General Motors.

Middle school years were highlighted by my winning the Catholic school city-wide spelling championship and later the city-wide essay contest. I was told that it was the first time any student in any school had finished first in both, though I cannot confirm that.

An important extracurricular activity began when our school started a Boy Scout troop, and I became immersed in scouting and remained very active in the troop until I got involved in athletics three years later. We competed in regional activities like building sleds to haul in a winter competition called the Klondike Derby. In the snow of Michigan this is not trivial.

Although at times it felt like we were in the Donner Party, the races ended with meals cooked around a welcome campfire, slightly better fare than the Donner Party cannibals had. (The Donner Party was a wagon train of American pioneers in the 1800s trapped by snow in the Sierra Nevada mountains on their way to California.) Other events in summer included racing in the Wagon Wheel Derby competition where bicycle tires supported a box-like covered structure that resembled a Conestoga wagon. We also hiked many trails which led to earning hiking medals and patches which we could proudly wear at regional events. One extended trip took us to five states in ten days, hiking more than 125 miles. This was my first trip away from home at age eleven and it made a lasting impression. It also taught me some self-reliance, particularly when our patrol got lost in the woods in another state. The scoutmaster wisely did not search for us but rather made us figure out how to get out of the woods on our own using compasses and a rudimentary map. Although we were not happy, it was a lesson well learned.

My scouting experience culminated in earning the Eagle Scout award with more than double the required merit badges. I had qualified at age twelve, but the national rules stipulated a recipient had to be age thirteen, so I continued that extra year, accumulating more merit badges. The troop kept us quite busy, a good thing for middle school-age boys. Little did I know that many years later after leaving scouting, I would be dragged back into the tent, so to speak, to serve on the board of directors of the National Eagle Scout Association (NESA).

About this time, I became dedicated to school athletics. I started playing football and basketball in 8th-grade and this carried on into high school at St. Matthew starting in 1965. We were a small Catholic school athletic power in Michigan, having won a state title a few years before. Now our high school team was loaded with talent, and we won consecutive state titles in basketball and an unofficial one in football though we were the top-rated team in our class in the state. Interestingly, my father Ted started on the only other back-to-back basketball state champions from Flint twenty-five years earlier.

One great example of community support occurred the day after we had won a very tough double overtime basketball game during the tournament. I was fouled after I stole the ball in the waning seconds of the tied game and scored to finally put us ahead. The next day, two burly police officers knocked on my front door. Although this might have been cause for concern on other days, I knew I had not done anything wrong lately.

My mother answered the door and the officers explained, "We are looking for Michael Manyak. We have a serious problem with him and have a warrant for his arrest."

As my mother blanched, I said they must be mistaken. They said no, it was for stealing the ball. That is what the citation said. The policemen had big grins as they delivered the warrant. The Flint police chief was the father of one of our team's cheerleaders. She was a good friend, and this was his way of congratulating me with his practical joke.

Many years later, when I was an adult, I was inducted into the Greater Flint Michigan Sports Hall of Fame in 1996 with my team, and the State of Michigan High School Athletic Association "Legends of the Game" in 2004. It was humbling and very gratifying to join my father in the Hall of Fame. These honors were unexpected so many years later, but it was great fun reconnecting with teammates, many of whom I had not seen in twenty-five years.

Along with my scouting activities and sports, I continued to excel in academics. I was the Salutatorian of my class and was a National Merit Semi-Finalist.

All told, Flint was a great place to grow up in the 1950s and 1960s with my sister Pat and brother Jim. There was financial stability with GM there at the time and we had a warm sense of community. It was now 1969 and I was graduating. It was time to leave my hometown and head to college.

I only applied to the University of Notre Dame where my father had gone on a baseball scholarship. Scholarships in athletics and for academic merit were mentioned when I interviewed but never materialized. The question of what to study was certainly influenced by my interest in biology. Though I still had an interest in paleontology, I really wanted to be in the field but understood that teaching would likely be a big part of that career. In my naivete, I did not know how they would be combined, so I elected to follow my interest in biology and went into the premedical program at Notre Dame. It was a small school with an undergraduate enrollment of around 5000 with students from all over the U.S. Little did I know that 1000 of the 1500 freshmen entrants would also select a premed curriculum. There was certainly increased competition with five percent of the Notre Dame freshman class who had been valedictorians of their high school class. Some of the tough science classes weeded out those not really interested and about 200 of us eventually graduated with a pre-med major and headed to medical or dental school.

But college was a time of many experiences, developing social skills and making lifelong friendships. One good memory was being a bartender at the post-game party of basketball coach Digger Phelps after we beat undefeated UCLA to end their 88-game winning streak, still the longest in history. The boisterous party included the president of Notre Dame, NBC executives, the Indiana governor, and other celebrities. They all came to the bartender, so I got to meet them. I have run into Digger a few times in later years and shared laughs when we were both signing our recently published books at exhibits in the Notre Dame bookstore.

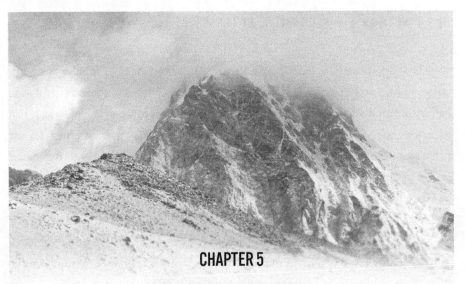

CHAPTER 5

RIDING THE RIG

A separate series of experiences influenced my decision about a career in medicine. My mother worked as a legal secretary and one of her firm's clients was the major ambulance company for the region. She mentioned to the client that I was going into premedical studies and the owner suggested that I come down and ride with the ambulances to get experience. I talked with the owner and staff. Although I did not have Emergency Medical Technician (EMT) training I had significant first aid training as an Eagle Scout. It turned out that the owner needed someone to cover the next evening shift and asked whether I would consider riding the rig with the most experienced ambulance attendant who was a highly respected first aid instructor in the county. Little did I know that when I agreed it would lead to some very vivid experiences that would solidify my interest in medicine as a career.

The first night I worked I had one of those calls that you cannot forget. After a few mundane calls that only required transporting people to the hospital, we received a call to be the second ambulance to the site of a shooting. I

29

quickly learned that if a second ambulance is summoned, the problem is significant and likely not pleasant. In this case, we learned after we arrived that a man
had committed suicide by shotgun to his head. We pulled up as the wife who had
witnessed the shooting was screaming hysterically as she was restrained on the
stretcher of the first ambulance which would take her for sedation and psychiatric
care. As she was taken away, we were left to clean up the suicide. The body had to
be taken to the hospital and the patient officially declared dead as a legal require-
ment. As I walked into the room, the body on the bed had no head. His face was
on his chest like a mask. Understandably, there was a copious amount of blood.
The worst part was when brain matter dripped from the ceiling onto my shoulder.
My experienced partner thought that he would never see me again. I did not sleep
well that night, still seeing what remained of the dead man's face, but I came back
the next weekend to work again, gaining the respect of my new colleagues.

I ended up not getting any scholarships for college, so I needed to work in
the summer and during school to help pay for my education. Right down the
street from Notre Dame campus was the McGann Funeral Home, a venerable
institution that also ran an ambulance that serviced the campus and surrounding
area, including portions of the Indiana Toll Road near campus. This was an ideal
opportunity because when I was on call at the funeral home, I could study. It was
not very busy at night as a funeral home, though occasionally there would be a
body in the room next to where I had to sleep at night, ever vigilant for strange
noises in the next room. However, I did have some memorable experiences in that
job. We received a call for a tanker gasoline truck explosion. We had to wait a
few hours until the fire died down to retrieve the driver who was horribly burned
and looked like a smoldering roast. Fires involving a fatality were very bad calls
because the smell was overpowering and difficult to wash off afterward.

A very entertaining time at the funeral home, if you will excuse the bad
visual image, were the stories from Grandpa McGann. This character had
founded the funeral home business and still came by periodically to make sure
things were in order. Grandpa McGann awed us with stories of the funeral of
legendary Notre Dame coach Knute Rockne, who still has the all-time highest
winning percentage in college football. Rockne and Gus Dorais had perfected
the forward pass in football at Notre Dame and used that for a famous upset of

Army in 1913. He had died at the peak of his career in a small plane crash in Kansas in 1931. The three days of funerary activities included a 200-limousine funeral procession at the height of the depression, attended by many political and celebrity figures and titans of business. Grandpa McGann also regaled us with stories about George Gipp, an All-American running back at Notre Dame in 1920. Gipp became famous for the statement he supposedly made to Coach Rockne on his deathbed about when the chips were down and the Irish were behind, to tell the team about him and tell them to "win one for the Gipper." The 1940 movie about Knute Rockne had Ronald Reagan as the young actor who played Gipp. Henceforth, Reagan was called The Gipper. According to Grandpa McGann, however, the Gipper wasn't quite a saint. He had contracted pneumonia while out partying for which he was well known. Apparently, it was quite a scene at the funeral when several gamblers and ladies of ill repute appeared to pay their respects. These stories sure made guys like Gipp seem more human and not enshrined on Mount Olympus.

Meanwhile, back in the summers in Flint, I continued to work on the ambulance and for Coca Cola, delivering products to stores. There were other tragic and crazy stories working on the ambulance, some dangerous and always unpredictable. One involved a high-speed multiple car accident in the county on a rainy night. We were first to arrive, and several cars were in a deep ditch and both cars and bodies were strewn throughout a field. There was lightning flashing in the pouring rain, gasoline was running down the street, and there were live wires jumping around. The first thing we had to do was assess who was most critical and who we could save while other ambulances were on the way. My partner was all of 130 pounds, and we had to lift the critical cases up a slippery, steep, 20-foot slope. We did get two victims up to our ambulance and got them to the hospital still alive but there ended up being several fatalities in that accident.

In another wreck, a young family was T-boned by a car which ran a stop sign at 70 mph. The father was decapitated and everyone else was dead, except a two-year-old boy. He was barely conscious, with a depressed skull fracture and was struggling to breathe because of facial fractures. He kept looking at me, his eyes pleading for me to help him. We made it to the hospital, but he did not survive. Many years later, I still tear up thinking about that little helpless child.

Occasionally I got to drive the ambulance on calls, though I preferred being the attendant. As the driver, you had even more responsibility for safety. This duty became very clear one night when I was working with one of my favorite ambulance partners who was also a stock car racer. I was home for Christmas from college, and he said we would alternate driving so I would get some experience driving on calls. The holiday crowd was in full force and traffic was quite congested. We received a call about a bad accident south of the city and my partner told me to drive. The strategy in traffic was to drive in the oncoming lane with full lights blazing and sirens blaring. Sure enough, some oblivious idiot pulled out into the oncoming lane right in front of us. With no time to decide at about 60 mph, my partner quickly yelled to stay off the brake. We had already discussed how braking could cause a skid and therefore a crash in a tight situation. We were on top of this car in a flash and I aimed for the narrow space between cars. I glanced sideways down as we whizzed by the cars and saw no space. We made it through, and my partner laughed very loudly and clapped me on the back, shouting "Great driving!" He told me he looked down on his side and could not see any space. I had done the same. We had made it through literally by inches. I started shaking after we stopped and did not stop for quite some time realizing the near miss which could very well have killed me. Fortunately, it was not my time.

Sometimes we had to navigate threats of violence at the scenes in high crime areas. We frequently were called by police but sometimes we were first on scene, though we tried to avoid that in high-crime areas. Sometimes we found ourselves in the middle of violence. One such situation occurred on a very busy day when all the other ambulances were out on runs.

Apparently, victim number one had been out all night in female company other than his wife and had been shot by his enraged spouse with a small caliber pistol when he returned. He retaliated by stabbing her and both were still going at each other when we arrived. They had now discarded their weapons and because all ambulances were tied up on other calls, we decided to load both patients in ours. This was not a good idea. No sooner had we started to go to the hospital than they started fighting again in the back of the ambulance. I had to jump between them to keep them from doing further harm. Fortunately, they did not injure me even though they still wanted to kill each other.

There were also some very hilarious times. One night we were called out on a sweltering night for someone having a seizure. The neighborhood was packed with people sitting on their porches trying to keep cool. An ambulance with lights and siren always draws considerable attention, none more than this night with everyone outside. A lady was on the second floor with very narrow stairs. As an option, there was an outdoor stairway that was visible to the neighborhood. When we assessed the situation, although we were not convinced that this was anything other than an event that involved alcohol and not a true seizure, we knew we had to take her in for evaluation if nothing more than to keep the neighborhood from getting upset. So, we decided to use the outdoor stairs as the most feasible method of evacuation. A huge crowd had gathered. Just as we bent down to pick up the stretcher with her on it, my partner split his pants wide open from front to back. His tighty-whities were now as clear as a beacon. He turned red as the whole crowd started to laugh. Of course, I was dying laughing, too. That made him even more mad, and he was using a profusion of multiple hyphenated curses directed at me, which made me laugh harder. We had to go down the very visible outside two flights like that with the crowd heckling him. When we got down, he took his outer ambulance shirt off and tied it around his waist. After all, we had to go to the hospital from there. Everyone at the hospital had a good chuckle as well.

One sleepy summer Sunday morning, we received a call that an old man had been found dead in his apartment and we needed to take him to the hospital to be pronounced. When we arrived at the old building, both the elevator and the stairs were too narrow for the stretcher. He was on the 8th floor, so we went to evaluate the situation, leaving our stretcher in the foyer. In his room, it was clear he had died several hours before and rigor mortis had set in. Fortunately, he was lying flat with his arms at his sides. He was literally as stiff as the proverbial board. Scratching our heads, we decided to put a large overcoat on him and put his fedora on along with his glasses. We thought we could bring him down upright and then place him on the stretcher at the ground level. We propped him up between us, grabbed his arms and frog-marched him to the elevator. Everything was fine until the elevator stopped on the 4th floor and a very old lady entered. We had his hat pulled low on his brow, but you could tell something was not right. We tried to keep a straight face and tried not to look at the lady. She was certainly startled when we came to the lobby and plopped the man on the stretcher. This happened three decades before a similar skit in the movie *Weekend At Bernie's*.

We never knew what circumstances we might face going on an ambulance call and sometimes had to be quite creative. That certainly was the case when we were called at McGann's to retrieve someone who had expired in a trailer. This guy was 750 pounds and died in the back bedroom. He was only thirty-four- years old but literally ate himself to death. We heard that he ate three dozen eggs for breakfast along with two pounds of bacon and a loaf of bread, and dinner was often four or five chickens. McGann's called me at my apartment to come in and help with the transport to the hospital. I recruited one of my roommates to help and it took eight of us to drag this guy out of the trailer once the door had been removed. The only vehicle that could accommodate him was the large Cadillac hearse at the funeral home which also was used as an ambulance. We had to leave the stretcher out and use a rug to transport him into the hearse. I stayed for the autopsy at the hospital and the pathologist had to cut through four feet of fat before the abdomen could be opened. He literally looked like a beached whale.

One had to prepare for the nauseating smells that accompanied finding a body which had decayed or after a bad burn. Sometimes placing a dab of mentholated petrolatum ointment like Vick's VapoRub™ under the nose helped but not always. For a decomposed body retrieval, often the best method of blocking the smell was to light up a nasty cigar. We always carried a cheap Italian brand of cigar in the ambulance that looked like a crooked rosebush stalk and smelled very strong though surprisingly did not taste too bad. Even that did not help when we found a homeless person who got locked in a railroad boxcar who was only found months later because of the smell and the buzz of the flies. As we retrieved the body, the head rolled off and had to be collected. This was so bad that we ran hot, meaning lights and siren, to the hospital with our heads out of the window. The cops at the hospital laughed at us until they got a whiff of the "patient." Even the crustiest, most experienced emergency personnel lost lunch over this one.

We also never knew when we would be thrust into a dangerous situation. One call from the police dispatcher involved a troublesome patient who needed to be transported to the hospital for evaluation. This could be anything from a psychotic episode to an overdose on psychotic street drugs. The important thing is to have police officers on site to control the scene. As I arrived at the top step of the porch, the door burst open, and a man ran full speed right at me. I had no choice but to go low and tackle him before he bulldozed me. He had thrown three large cops and made a dash for freedom just as we got there. I got him down and the police piled on him and finally subdued him. He certainly appeared to be on some illegal pharmaceutical.

Working the ambulance over Christmas vacation from college, we were called to the large auditorium in Flint to get a patient at the national Weatherman War Council. This was an American militant organization that carried out a series of domestic terrorism activities from 1969 through the 1970s which included bombings, jailbreaks, and riots. This meeting changed them into an underground organization that would commit strategic acts of sabotage against the government. Police were not allowed into the auditorium occupied by hundreds of radicals, but we were allowed entry since we were providing help. This was covered by national news for several days and we were shown bringing out a patient headed to the hospital.

Sometimes we were rewarded for our work with gratitude. I remember very well the man who walked into the McGann funeral home asking for the guys who had extracted him from a bad car wreck. This had occurred six months before in mid-December on a cold night when we were called to the scene of a one-car wreck where the vehicle was upside down and the driver trapped. We could not reach inside to remove him. As we waited for police and a tow truck to get the car upright, I noted that the driver was bleeding profusely from a large scalp laceration. I decided, perhaps foolishly, that we had better do something or he would die from blood loss. I had my partner stabilize the car and I took hemostats and bandages and crawled upside down under the car. If the car had shifted, I could have been crushed but I really did not think about that, this guy was dying in front of my eyes. Through the broken windshield I was able to use the hemostats to stop some of the bleeding and created pressure bandages that I could wrap around his head. Fortunately, the bleeding was controlled, and I crawled out from under the car.

Now that he was out of the hospital and recovered, he had come to thank us personally and brought his skull x-rays that showed about a six-inch linear posterior skull fracture. He was profusely thankful. The personal satisfaction for doing the right thing even though seemingly crazy cannot be matched, never mind that I violated the cardinal rule of responders to make sure you are safe first. I had just reacted and not thought. This type of follow up gratitude was rare, but it sure made me feel that the job was worth it. The look on his face was priceless. Frankly, this type of experience of truly helping someone in need solidified my desire to be a physician and surgeon.

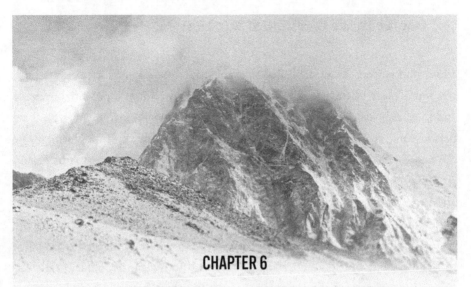

CHAPTER 6

JOHNSON & JOHNSON: CORPORATE MEDICAL SALES BEFORE MEDICAL SCHOOL

While I was waiting to hear from medical school, I returned to Flint and lived with my parents, which wasn't ideal for me or them. I needed to earn some money, so I interviewed for an introductory sales job with a modest salary and commission for a pharmaceutical company. However, I was hired by the recruitment company to work for them even though I had no experience.

One early lesson I learned by observation was some managers had favorable impressions of someone who resembled them. I was given a list of contact leads of district managers for pharmaceutical companies. Managers are always looking for good people so are open to being contacted about potential candidates. My strategy was to present four candidates. The first would be not your strongest candidate but someone who did fit the requirements. The second candidate was a rock star, an IBM or medical device sales rep who was clearly overqualified. This would have the manager drooling over the prospect even though he could not afford that person. This established that you could identify quality candidates. It was not a waste of time for the candidates who viewed it as a potential upgrade and sales reps always listen to the possibility of a job improvement. The third person you put in front of the manager would be the one you thought might be the best fit and was really the one you wanted to place. Frequently, this person was a successful sales rep in perhaps a more entry level position or a company with a less prestigious type of product. The fourth candidate would be someone not as qualified but still in the ballpark with credentials. The added benefit of being successful was that if you placed someone already working in another company, that company then had an opening. The obvious move was to contact that company with a vacancy at the appropriate time. Therefore, you churned the pot and created potential business.

Consequently, I met many pharmaceutical district sales managers. They would ask about my background and nearly every manager would ask if I was interested in the job. I was now on the waiting list for acceptance into Indiana University and University of Michigan medical schools. These were not guarantees of admission and I felt it was necessary to consider a career in medical sales and management as an attractive fallback career position. I had multiple offers and took the position offered by Johnson & Johnson (J & J). Once I accepted, they told me I was the next person to receive a territory in the continental U.S. I had visions of rural Montana or Appalachia and was surprised when they called, and somewhat apologetically, told me that the territory in southwestern Michigan and northern Indiana was mine. Since I grew up in Michigan and went to school in northern Indiana, this was more attractive than they imagined. They told me previous sales reps had considered Fort Wayne, Indiana, to be the best city to live in but that South Bend was also an option. I told them I thought it was time to expand business in the South Bend area. I was excited; I was going back one year after graduating from Notre Dame but this time with a job and income.

The years at J&J were invaluable because I learned a good deal about the business end of medicine, experience that would stand me in good stead in future years. The training program was extensive and highly respected in the industry. Furthermore, my regional manager was one of the most beloved managers in the entire company and I remember him very fondly for his guidance and friendship.

He claimed for years the best time he had visiting a sales rep was when he came to South Bend and we went to a barbecue joint instead of the usual steak dinner. The older African American owner was hilarious and we had a great time listening to his stories. We proceeded from there to a local pub to shoot pool with several Notre Dame football players there for the summer practice sessions. As a diehard Ohio State alum and fan, he thoroughly loved meeting them. We did not talk much business that night but sure had a good time.

While I was growing the business in the territory, I still had not given up on med school. My mom's brother, an attorney, was married to a Filipino nurse who taught at the University of Michigan. My aunt suggested I consider med school in the Philippines; she had two brothers who were doctors educated there. This was a very attractive option as I learned more. I am forever indebted to my aunt and uncle for encouraging me to go to the Philippines because it dramatically changed my life.

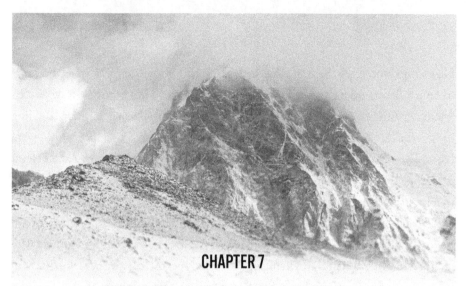

CHAPTER 7

A FASCINATING OPPORTUNITY
IN THE ASIAN TROPICS

E ven though the Philippines has more than 7000 islands and 78 dialects, the language of instruction had been English since the U.S. had acquired the islands at the turn of the 20th century from Spain. The textbooks were the same as those used in U.S. medical schools, and most of the professors had been trained in the States. Students also received extensive hands-on experience in the clinics unlike many other foreign and U. S. medical schools.

My aunt's sister and her attorney husband held mid-level government positions in the Philippines, and she delivered my application to the medical school that seemed best for me, University of the East. However, I still needed a comparative anatomy class to be accepted. Fortunately, I was able to take that in the graduate school of biology at Notre Dame over the summer. It was quite intense because I had to go to the lab when I was finished with my job and work for several hours more each night. I was the only one there most nights and I had my own key. My boss at J&J was very helpful because the company paid for the class under the pretense that anatomical knowledge was beneficial to understand the product usage. Once I completed this class, I was accepted into medical school. I closed my career at J&J, but those experiences were instrumental in progressing my medical career and gave me a greater understanding of the business side of medicine. It also gave me respect for what sales reps had to go through to see physicians at hospitals. While many physicians refuse to see sales reps, once I was a practicing physician, out of respect for their efforts, I set aside time to see them if they made an appointment.

So, as a recent premed college grad but now with experience in the real world, I packed a tropical wardrobe in 1975 and flew to Manila, Philippines, to attend the University of the East Ramon Magsaysay Memorial Medical Center (UERM). My preconceived ideas of studying in an oceanside bamboo hut and diving in the ocean after lunching on coconuts and papaya were blown away as soon as I landed. The densely populated capital city had over 20 million people concentrated on Manila Bay. I had expected something more resort tropical. It was tropical all right, steaming hot and humid but it was a crazy vibrant city all lit up in bright lights.

I arrived during the height of martial law imposed by then President Ferdinand Marcos who lifted martial law at the end of my second year there. It was a race to get home during martial law though we avoided that mostly by starting the evening early. With the repeal of martial law Manila was open all night and it was like the wild west. Good thing I usually had to be up early to keep temptation at bay!

The UERM medical school was comprised of classrooms in two or three buildings but as expected in a developing country, resources were scarce. The hallways were not air conditioned. There were regular electrical interruptions which made it difficult to concentrate in the sweltering tropical climate. The air was quite polluted with constant fumes from exhaust in crowded Manila. We wore tailor-made white uniforms. Tailors and cloth were cheap with an added advantage that uniformity eliminated distinction between wealthy and people with less means. Amenities you took for granted in the States might not be available. One lesson learned quickly was that there were no toilet seats and worse, no toilet paper, in public toilets.... but also, in the medical school. The latter was probably true because the toilet paper would be stolen. We all carried some tissues for gastrointestinal emergencies which occurred with regularity in this country where water and food could be contaminated.

There is always an adjustment ascending to the next level of academics and this was certainly true of medical school where all classes were now science-oriented, and you had to learn a new language of medicine. A full day of various classes was followed by significant reading in preparation for the next day. There was no shortcut for the sheer volume of studies. Believe me, we all looked for ways to shorten the days or absorb knowledge more efficiently. The first year was comprised primarily of basic sciences like biochemistry, anatomy, and physiology; in the second and third years we tied basic sciences to clinical application in pathology and public health classes. The fourth year was all clinical experience as we rotated through various disciplines including surgery, obstetrics and gynecology, and emergency medicine. We were still expected to study during the exhausting clinical rotations.

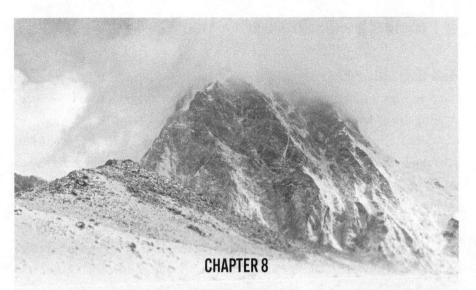

CHAPTER 8

CADAVERS IN CLASSROOMS, COLLEGE AND PRO HOOPS, AND A CHRISTMAS CAROL

The first year was particularly memorable for the anatomy lab. We were divided into lab groups of ten students and each group was assigned a cadaver to be dissected over the course of the year. The cadavers were preserved in formalin and stored in a tank and then put on a large table. We never knew where the cadavers came from and speculated that they were prisoners who had died (one had a sling still on his broken arm). In the beginning, despite the initial distaste of working on a dead body that reeked of formalin preservative, structures could be readily identified as we meticulously dissected the tissues. When the lab was finished, the lab techs would put a tarpaulin over the body and leave it on the table for the next day. Well, as you can imagine, you could smell the anatomy lab located on the fourth floor as you entered the building at ground level. This was compounded in the tropical climate where the lab windows were left open. Furthermore, we frequently had to shoo feral cats off the bodies as we came in and found them chewing on some body part. By the second semester, the bodies had shriveled, making dissection more difficult.

Tests were often plagued by problems not usually found in U. S. medical schools. The class of about 200 students was divided into three different sections and we were all herded into one big classroom. One section was allowed to take the test first while the other groups had to remain in the classroom to discourage any sharing of answers with the next section. The third section had to wait for the other two to finish which could take four hours, during which the last student section became anxious and bored. For one test, I was in the third section, and we had waited several hours for our turn. Just after we started our lab practical, a tropical depression storm struck with buckets of rain, strong wind, and floods. The electricity went out, as frequently happens. But the show must go on. We now had to aim our microscope mirrors at the window where there was dull ambient light instead of the microscope light.

You simply had to roll with the punches. One particularly vocal student who always complained was in front of me at a station that required us to look at an x-ray to determine the pathology. As the storm raged and the lights remained out, we had about thirty seconds to answer the question at each station and then had to move to the next. With the lights out we had to take an x-ray to the window to look at it. Right when he held it up, a strong gust of wind whipped the film out of his hand and blew it 10 feet away. He screamed and cursed while he ran to retrieve it. Just when he got to it, the bell rang to move to the next station. He went apoplectic, jumping up and down, screaming and cursing like Donald Duck in a cartoon. It was hilarious and I was laughing so hard I almost missed the next question. His antics certainly broke the tension.

Anatomy lab tests could be perplexing as the cadavers shriveled over the year. There were fifty stations set up with microscopes with slides or some anatomical structure to identify. Halfway into a test later in the year one station had a desiccated globular structure with a pin in it that said "Identify". I had no idea what this was and comparing notes with other students when we finished there were a variety of guesses. One said it was an eyeball, another said it was a testicle, another thought it was an ovary. Who knew? I was convinced I had to be more of a forensic anthropologist than a physician for some of these items.

I was fortunate that when I first arrived, I was able to live with my aunt's sister in a Manila suburb. The family was very generous but also very protective and the door was locked at 9 p.m. After a few months, I decided to move in with an American classmate to an apartment in a working-class neighborhood, replete with chickens, street vendors, and lots of ambient noise. My aunt's sister had an ornate Roman-style marble bathtub with brass fixtures. We got the idea to take a photo in it individually and make Christmas cards. No one back home had any idea about life in the Philippines and likely had the same misconceptions that I had originally had about it being like Gilligan's Island instead of a huge vibrant city. My aunt's Filipino American nephew lived with her temporarily; he was a U.S. college student and avid amateur photographer. I coerced my very attractive classmate girlfriend to sit on my lap in her bathing suit while lighting a cigar for me for the photo in the bathtub. We had some props of a paper mâché Santa and a surgical textbook and I got the perfect photo with the cigar lit and us laughing. More than four decades later, I still hear from my friends about that memorable card. One friend in Notre Dame law school opened my card while in class and shared it with the professor and classmates on a bleak snowy day and everybody had a good laugh. That was the overwhelming response to the card with one notable exception.... my parents. They wanted to see me with a stethoscope and white coat examining a patient, not a bikini-clad beauty, never mind that she was a Harvard grad and top medical student.

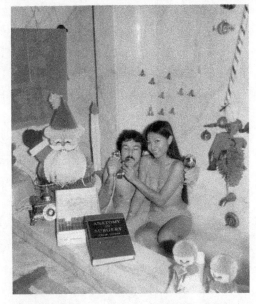

Christmas card from the Philippines in marble Roman bathtub.

Another interesting event occurred near the end of my first year. The heavyweight boxing championship of the world was held in Manila. This became one of the greatest fights of all time with Muhammed Ali versus Joe Frazier, a bruising 14 round fight held in the largest coliseum in Manila. Since the tickets were very costly, we watched a close circuit broadcast of the brutal fight (along with an estimated billion others around the world) which was stopped after the 14th round when Frazier conceded.

The day after the fight I had tickets for a Temptations concert and was curious why six seats right in front of us were empty. Right at the start of the concert, in walked Muhammed Ali and his entourage and he sat right in front of me. His head was swollen like a pumpkin, and he was still obviously in pain.

Even though the Americans brought some of our culture to the Philippines, it was still quite a shock to learn that basketball was hugely popular there. Tennis, golf, soccer, and to a lesser extent baseball were also sports played in the Philippines but basketball was far and away the most popular. The pro league regularly played to capacity crowds in large arenas. The University Athletic Association of the Philippines (UAAP) was the collegiate equivalent of the NCAA in the US and UE was a member. I had a fortuitous opportunity to scrimmage against the college varsity and the coach asked me to play for the team.

The UE Warriors were reigning UAAP champions. We practiced right at the gym right on the medical school campus. Filipino basketball players are shorter and lighter than American college players, but they could shoot well and were fast. The UE coach was a well-known former big basketball star and the UE athletic director was also the pro coach of the top team in the professional league and sometimes he would bring the team to practice at the same gym. It created quite a buzz on the campus because these players were celebrities and very well known nationally. They always attracted quite a crowd to watch them practice which usually numbered several hundred fans.

It was quite an honor that the pro coach who often watched our practices asked me to join the practices with the pro team. The pro league rules stipulated that each team could have two "imports" per season, so all teams tried to get tall U.S. basketball players with college or pro experience. The coach told me he was trying to get me classified as a Filipino citizen because I lived there the whole year, and therefore would not count as one of the imports. The league officials, however, overruled that idea and I was relegated to practice only. For two years I played on the UE team every week on national tv in front of a crowd of 16,000 fans. For several years after playing, I would meet Filipinos who remembered me playing.

One day our athletic director (and pro coach) came to me to see if I had any big basketball player friends back in the U.S. who might be good enough and who would consider playing in the pro league. I contacted Digger Phelps, the coach at Notre Dame, and found out that to see if there were any players not playing somewhere who might be available. Pete Crotty, a 6-foot 9-inch forward, was not playing anywhere after a pro basketball job in Sweden had fallen through. I knew Pete rather well and he would be perfect for this team laden with Filipino stars. Pete was a perfect fit because his strengths of rebounding and defense complemented the Filipino players who were good shooters, but also because he was very friendly and would mesh with his teammates.

When Pete arrived, the pro coach and I went straight to one of the pro games in progress. Members of the press noticed Pete, congregated around him, and had an impromptu press conference. This was quite amusing since they thought I was his agent and they asked me questions as well. We laughed and winged it and the press wrote about Pete's introduction to the pro basketball scene in Manila.

The pro team went on to win the pro league championship over the next several months. Trying to keep a low profile at school, my cover was blown at one game when a big fight broke out in the stands right in front of us behind the bench. Filipinos like to gamble, and significant money was wagered on basketball in addition to other things like cock fights. There would be angry claims of collusion if the referees made a questionable or outright bad call. These angry fans would throw coins on the floor or other hard items making it dangerous to be on the court. One particularly raucous evening the fans got in an argument and started throwing chairs. A photographer snapped a photo that appeared on the front page of the largest paper and there we were right in the middle of the photo, very easily identified fans. So much for staying low key.

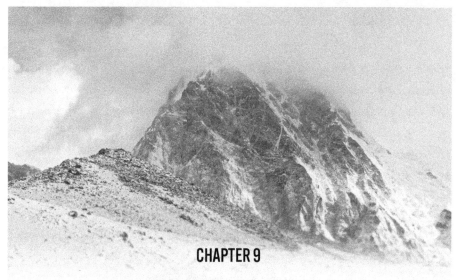

CHAPTER 9

MONKEYSHINES

About this time, I moved into an apartment with a small yard close to school and acquired a pet monkey, the most amazing pet I have ever had. Monkeys are indeed among the most fascinating mammals, no doubt due to their human-like features and obvious intelligence. Monkeys are incredibly strong for their size and can deliver a vicious bite which, if it breaks the skin, must be treated as an infected wound. Furthermore, they can carry bacterial and viral diseases that affect humans, including TB and hepatitis but not rabies.

My pet monkey was a crab-eating macaque native to the Philippines. It was a great companion but required constant surveillance and needed attention. Slightly larger than a squirrel and smart as a whip, it had the agility of an NBA basketball guard and curiosity of a two-year old child, a dangerous combination, so you always had to be on your toes.

I acquired the monkey at the end of my first year when I attended a party with ex-pats and one of them was returning to the U.S. and could not take the monkey. She was still quite young and had not cut her permanent adult teeth. I renamed her Juju after the Hausa (African) language term for "fetish" or "evil spirit" which was used in the old Tarzan movies. Although not an African monkey, I felt the name would likely be a good fit because she was quite mischievous. I kept her outside with a dog chain around her waist, so she had freedom of movement between two palm trees along a ten-foot bamboo pole with a small house to sleep in at one end like a bird house but larger. Juju was one tough customer and feral cats and large rats the size of raccoons would not bother her.

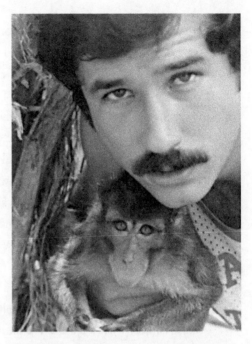

Juju the crab-eating macaque, the most entertaining pet, who had the inquisitiveness of a two-year-old child and agility of an NBA guard.

Very affectionate with me and the maid, Juju was wary but indifferent to most friends and highly protective against strangers. The one exception was my friend the veterinary student who graciously supplied important vaccinations for Juju for the price of a good dinner and a few drinks. She did not like him.

Juju could pry or tear just about anything apart and particularly loved mango seeds which she ripped apart to get the kernel. She could be very destructive if left loose to her own curiosity. This agility could be beneficial, however. I will never forget the night the electricity was off and the heat unbearable, so much so that I decided to brave the clouds of mosquitoes outside. I brought the monkey and she sat on my shoulder and caught any mosquitoes that came close. Her night vision was exquisite. How about that for environmentally friendly mosquito protection!

Juju had figured out how to open her small lock by peeling a palm frond to make a tool and jimmying the lock. Originally, I had her on a dog chain that had the hand-operated clasp, but I watched her grasp that like a human and open the clasp. Juju basically had four hands with opposable thumbs and a prehensile tail.

If she got loose, which she did on occasion, it would take patience and a piece of banana to get her back. I had the maid purchase a small padlock with a key. About two weeks later, Juju was out in the yard again. We finally got her back on her chain but then found her out soon again. We coerced her back after some time and decided to watch around the corner. She waited until we had gone and then we saw her take a running leap at the palm tree and just barely pull a frond down which she proceeded to strip and make a stick. She then grabbed the small padlock and jimmied the lock open. Wow! If I had not seen that I would not have believed it. Obviously, we had to escalate the security. I had the maid get a combination lock. Fortunately, she could not open that despite trying to turn the dial as she had seen us working the lock. What an amazing pet!

Monkey-human encounters are legendary. A friend was in a travel lodge in Zambia with signs saying to look out before opening the door. The local monkeys had learned how to knock on the door like the maids and would rush into the room when the tourist opened it, trashing the place and stealing food and clothing. In Cambodia, tourists are warned not to feed the monkeys. According to an eyewitness, one tourist had a cup of nuts in one hand while offering one nut with the other. The monkey went to get the single nut but suddenly smacked the guy in the face and grabbed the whole cup. He was stunned and could not react. Nothing like getting mugged by a monkey! Special forces friends tell a very funny story about advancing in full battle gear with drawn automatic weapons on a purportedly abandoned Central American villa previously owned by a drug lord. While they were debating about how to breach the door, a monkey came running out of the brush suddenly, scampered up to the door, opened it, and stood there like a doorman. He had been trained to open the door!

Monkeys are amazing animals. I do believe Juju was smarter than at least half the people I knew. Those little monkeys are more than a match for the pickpockets in Rome or Rio. Just like with human pickpockets, beware of groups!

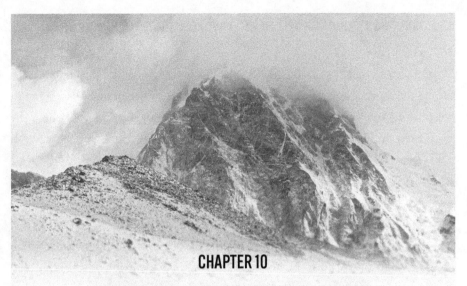

CHAPTER 10

TROPICAL TRANSPORTATION

When I first arrived, we traveled to the city and school in taxis, in tricycles with side cars like Vietnamese tuk-tuks, or in small open back jeeps called jeepneys that followed routes and made stops like a bus in the States. Buses were also available but were really crowded and spewed dark exhaust pollution, so we usually avoided them. Even though taxis and other public transportation were abundant and not expensive, most of us eventually purchased cars.

I acquired a partially rusted-out old tank of a 1960 diesel Mercedes. This old clunker was notorious for stranding me and tended to break down just about as far away from home as possible.

The only time the car came through in the clutch was once when I was downtown, and a typhoon was on the way. I had joined a close friend at our local watering hole and was not paying close attention to the coming storm. We went to the door and the water was up to the third step. I decided to make a run for it in the hope I would not be stranded for a couple of days. I literally ran in driving rain and strong wind a couple of blocks to where I was parked on Manila Bay.

Since these old diesels started with a glow plug that then ignited the engine, once the engine started it would run in all kinds of weather. Certain that I was going to be stranded and would end up staying overnight in a bar, I could not believe the car started in this raging storm. It was like driving a boat on the way home with a wake behind me but more dangerous because craters in the road could not be detected. But for once the bomb made it and I gratefully slept in my own bed. It was a happy day when I left this mechanical abomination behind when I left the country a few years later.

Driving in Manila was quite an experience. Frankly, all one needed was a steering wheel and a horn, brakes were optional. People ran lights all the time. The only thing a working traffic light signified is that there was electricity in that area. You really needed to pay attention. Surprisingly, there were relatively few accidents for the intense volume of the crazy traffic. This was very surprising since the drivers routinely made six lanes out of four. At a red light, when they did stop, the drivers would all creep and begin an all-out race at the green light. Any pedestrians in the road had to run for their lives.

Driving at night was like going on a safari. You never knew what you would encounter on the roads. Lighting was sporadic. Vehicles were driven on the wrong side of the divided highways, and you had to dodge pedestrians running across the road and avoid large craters with no warning signs that could break the axle. Dangerous obstacles ranged from broken-down vehicles just abandoned, to buses cutting you off, or the occasional water buffalo plodding down the middle of the road.

Despite the suffocating heat, hordes of people, treacherous transportation, and quirks of culture and nature, I was now accustomed to life in the tropics and starting to enjoy it. I read about a paralyzing blizzard back in Michigan while I was in cutoff shorts and tank top with my maid cooking dinner. I decided then I was not going back to live in Michigan. After all, I had a maid, pet monkey, an old Mercedes (however misleading in significance), and was going scuba diving on the weekend. This was all in addition to getting a great education. Going to the Philippines turned out to be the best move I ever made.

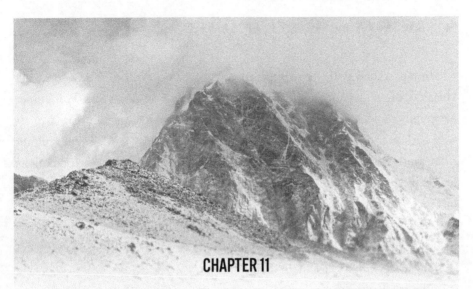

CHAPTER 11

A PROFUSION OF PARASITES AND POVERTY

B ack in the clinics, my education continued unabated. We would often see x-rays of patients with giant worms and other such parasites. A parasite adapted to human temperatures so when a patient underwent anesthesia for a procedure where their temperature was often lowered, the worms would think that the patient was dying and escape from their noses and mouths. The president of our class and close friend Joey Mendieta, who completed part of his training in Manila, was a surgical resident in the operating room when the surgeon operating on a patient with intestinal obstruction extracted a large earthworm-sized parasitic round worm. But there were more, and he kept pulling out worm after worm, all squirming, and put them into a large pan. When it became full, he handed the disgusting, wriggling mess to the nurse to dispose of it but she shrieked and threw the pan into the air, spilling all the worms into the open abdominal cavity, to the horror of all in the operating room. That required meticulous extraction of each segment with thorough irrigation to prevent seeding the abdominal cavity with parasites, adding a couple of hours to the case.

In our second year, we worked in an indigent ob-gyn hospital, Jose Fabella Hospital, often in 12-hour shifts. The hospital is ground zero of the Philippines' overpopulation crisis and more than 50,000 babies are delivered a year. Women were packed two to a bed, head to foot. As medical students, we delivered children from mothers who had previous children and the residents delivered mothers' first babies or if a baby was in breach position. It was like a production line of births. Once delivered, the placentae were then put in a large plastic bin to be sent to have human chorionic gonadotropin hormone extracted. But in this very poor hospital, you had to keep the lid on the bin because you would see stray cats slinking away with a placenta in their mouth.

The mother often needed to have a small incision called an episiotomy to allow the baby's head to emerge because the women were quite small. We would then suture this closed, using absorbable suture. Supplies were in short demand, so any leftover suture material was placed in a boiling pot to sterilize it for the next person.

Those women who needed dilation and curettage (D & C) were lined up five at a time with no screens between their beds and the scraping procedures were performed sequentially to remove retained placental fragments from the uterus.

In the fourth year, we rotated through different services. One rotation was the infectious disease center of the Philippines, San Lazaro. We were assigned in groups of ten and my first assignment was to the cholera ward. Cholera is a bacterial gastrointestinal infection that causes copious diarrhea and is survivable if you vigorously replace the fluids and electrolytes lost. Antibiotics are also used but fluid and electrolyte replacement are key. As we received our orientation, I noted patients on cots with holes in the bottom having projectile diarrhea while shivering violently with wide open intravenous fluids going in every extremity. It looked like a scene from an old horror movie. As I wondered how the large bed-pans now beginning to overflow were going to be emptied, a nurse's aide shuffled over nonchalantly, picked up a pan without gloves, and wrestled it to the open window where she proceeded to empty it.

All I could think was that I was going to die here!

The diphtheria section wasn't much more comforting. The diphtheria bacteria create a film across the back of the throat and the patient suffocates if not treated. You must keep the airway open. We were fortunate to have a world expert on diphtheria, a woman about five feet tall who was quite humorous. When she started with us, she declared loudly, "I AM THE DIPHTHERIA BACILLUS!" She got our attention for sure. We followed her on rounds as she pulled the jaws of patients open and poked her index finger through the pseudomembrane blocking the airway without gloves as she went from patient to patient.

The tetanus section was filled with end stage patients, too. This bacterium caused painful muscle contractions particularly to the head and neck, so it's sometimes called lockjaw. The patients suffered from opisthotonos, severe muscle spasms triggered by loud noises, so if we clapped our hands, they would go into spasms.

The TB Sanitorium of the Philippines, the national referral center, looked like the images you've seen of a concentration camp. Tuberculosis was called consumption because the patients just waste away and look like cadavers ambling slowly around the facility. TB can mimic many medical conditions and can appear in any area of the body. I learned that if you could diagnose TB, you would become a good doctor because it mimicked so many other things. This was another disease I was afraid of contracting. All this training would come to be used in various ways. In fact, TB is currently on the upswing in the world with antibiotic resistant strains.

The Philippines is a hot bed of infectious diseases. There are three strains of malaria, filariasis (potentially causing elephantiasis), leptospirosis every time there was a flood, and amebic dysentery is rampant. You can get serious diarrhea from any number of bacteria and one-celled organisms. Schistosomiasis carried by snails and large liver flukes can attack your liver. Dengue fever and chikungunya are endemic.

The national pediatric hospital was a sad place for me. Babies were abandoned by their parents because of poverty. Many of them suffered from kwashiorkor, a protein malnutrition which caused them to be very thin with poor integrity of their blood vessels and a bloated belly. We would have to put a tiny butterfly needle into their scalp veins if we could. If we did not get fluid into them, they would die. I spent a week at the emergency room there where I sat in a folding chair overnight. Watching the sick children was difficult and cured me of any desire to pursue pediatrics.

I also hated the charity neurology ward. There were no respirators so if a patient was in a coma, two med students would have to use a portable manual ventilator to get air into the lungs. We took ten-minute turns physically pumping air through a mask over the patients' mouth and nose to facilitate breathing. It was utterly exhausting.

One time during school, I got violently ill with fluids coming out of both ends and a high fever making me delirious. I didn't go to the hospital to work for three days and lost thirteen pounds the hard way. I was seriously dehydrated when my maid came in and said she would get me some medicine from the local sari-sari store, a small convenience store that doubled as a rudimentary pharmacy. For pennies she brought some black Alka Seltzer-like tablets. The tablets contained activated charcoal to soak up toxins, atropine which is a very powerful nerve blocking agent to shut down the bowels, and a sulfa antibiotic to kill many types of bacteria. These reversed my condition within a few hours and were a godsend. These miracle pills would not be legal in the U.S., but I traveled with them all the time for years afterwards.

My experience with tropical diseases proved helpful later. During my internship in New York, an elderly man who had never left New York had what looked like liver cancer. But I suggested that he be tested for amebae, a parasite that can cause an abscess, because the lesion had a smooth periphery not usually seen in cancer. Although ridiculed by all but the chief resident, it turned out that the patient tested positive for amebae. The chief resident was thrilled when he came with a big grin on his face to tell me I had been right. Instead of unnecessary surgery, he was treated with antiparasitic medicine. No one had seen this before, but I had.

Another time, my close friend Russell Wright called me about his Indiana friend visiting Washington with his nationally ranked junior tennis player son. The son had a bad case of diarrhea and abdominal pain and had to withdraw from the tournament when the antibiotic he had been prescribed did not work. I told them that the antibiotic would have helped if he had a bacterial infection. I called in a prescription for a different medication used for protozoan (one-celled organisms) infection. This could be amebic or more likely something called giardia which is found in freshwater streams and ponds. The ecstatic father called me twelve hours later saying the symptoms were gone and thanked me profusely.

My experience with tropical diseases and remote expeditions prompted Peter Hotez, then GW Chairman of the Department of Immunology, Microbiology, and Tropical Medicine and now Founding Dean of the US National School of Tropical Medicine, to offer a position as professor in his department. It was a great honor that I held for ten years.

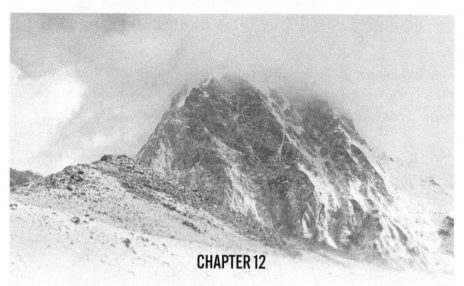

CHAPTER 12

VIOLENT STORMS AND VOLCANOES

The threat of death by infectious diseases was only one major cause for concern in the Philippines. One of the other vagaries of living in the tropics was the uncertainty of violent weather. Basically, there are two seasons in the Philippines, Rainy Season and Not Rainy Season. It was always hot and very humid except for January and February. In the rainy season, the humidity ranged from 90 to 100 percent. Nearly daily rains began in July and extended to December. The rains often caused flooding, particularly in low-lying areas with poor drainage near the rivers. What really got everyone excited was the occurrence of a typhoon, a powerful cyclonic storm. The only difference between a hurricane and a typhoon is the location where the storm occurs. Hurricane is used to describe these storms in the North Atlantic and central and eastern North Pacific. The same type of disturbance in the Northwest and South Pacific is called a typhoon while it is a cyclone in South Asia.

Usually, you had a few days advance warning that a typhoon was coming. It was advisable to stock up on potable water by filling large garbage cans, collect food to last at least a week, as well as candles, matches, batteries, flashlights, and books to read. Typhoon parties sprung up as people readied to be sequestered for several days without electricity. I learned early to take this warning seriously. I was stranded for two days in my first year, fortunately in an apartment building with friends but supplies ran low before we waded out of the building.

Typhoons are incredibly destructive, and they are graded like hurricanes with Category 1 to 5 increasing with increased wind velocity. Thus, news of a high category typhoon headed toward Manila created a lot of anxiety in October 1978 during my fourth year when we were in our clinical rotations. Making the usual preparations in earnest, we still had time for a few typhoon parties.

As the storm came closer it intensified such that it was predicted to be Category 5 when it hit Manila. We decided that the monkey would have to come inside to protect her. It required serious surveillance to keep an eye on her in the laundry room, to keep her out of the living area. As the storm intensified, we now had significant concern as we battened down the hatches. At about 10:30 pm the electricity went out as Metro Manila authorities tried to minimize the expected damage from live wires. We could hear the storm approaching, sounding like a freight train. It struck Manila 30 minutes later with violent ferocity and winds of 220 kilometers per hour (140 mph). The two large palm trees in my front yard were blown parallel to the ground like in the movies. Debris was flying through the air. It looked like the end of the world. Fortunately, my apartment was at ground level in a very solid large complex house which was significantly elevated from the nearby riverbank. This elevation was a good thing because the floods ended up reaching the front of my yard.

This typhoon was classified a super typhoon and named Typhoon Tip or Typhoon Warling in the Philippines. Today It is still the largest tropical cyclone ever recorded anywhere with a diameter of 1380 miles. The 2013 Super Typhoon Haiyan that hit the Philippines supposedly had sustained winds above 150 mph but smaller diameter. These storms took several lives and weeks for the floods to subside.

Residual effects from these types of storms had an impact in the clinics. Because of the polluted water flooding, there were outbreaks of hepatitis, gastroenteritis, and other water-borne diseases such as typhoid. Leptospirosis, a bacterial disease passed in rat urine into the water supply, causes high fever, headaches, vomiting, muscle aches, and jaundice along with a characteristic rash. There was always an increase in hospital admissions after a flood due to these diseases.

Mother Nature could be incredibly violent in the Philippines, frequently making whimsical appearances without warning. In my time there, I weathered three moderate earthquakes which were alarming but with few injuries and correspondingly moderate damage. In my second year there the volcano in the center of Lake Taal, a recreational lake about two hours outside of Manila, began to erupt with smoke appearing from the cone. I had never seen an active volcano so two of us left before curfew was lifted at 4 a.m. to view this natural phenomenon. Driving through the provinces in the dark in a jeep with a hole in the muffler, we arrived just after dawn at the tourist lodge overlooking the lake. There it was, Taal volcano spewing long columns of smoky debris 8,000 feet in the air. We ate breakfast and watched the show before leaving in the early afternoon. It turned out that was the only day the eruption was visible; the rest of the week it rained, and visibility was poor.

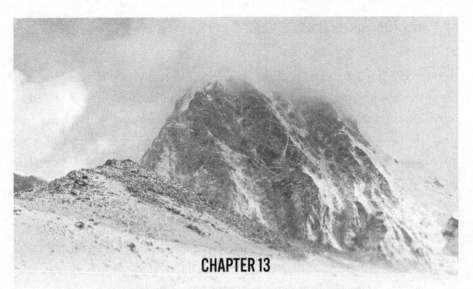

CHAPTER 13

HOBBITS AND CHRISTMAS

The huge typhoon passed, and, in its wake, life resumed though it was a few months until things were back to normal.

My favorite place was The Hobbit House which opened midway during our medical stint. The place was based on the Tolkien series later made famous in movies. But in a uniquely Filipino way, the owner expat Jim Turner hired Filipino dwarves as staff, so all waiters, bartenders, and bouncers were "hobbits". Before you condemn this practice, you must understand that these people were resigned to the lowest rungs of society with few chances for work. So, Jim Turner gave them employment. Over the course of several years, he made them the managers and turned the establishment over to them as owners. They loved him for it.

The first night I was there after its recent opening, it was quite crowded, and they had a great band. Filipinos are talented musicians and can copy any style of music and they speak great English. They are frequently entertainers throughout Asia. I kept feeling like someone was walking past me but just thought I was being jostled by customers. Finally, I looked down and the waiters were passing through the forest of legs delivering drinks. It was hilariously clever. I had not known the owner had hired dwarves. It became a regular hangout for several of us and I was especially pleased to learn that Jim Turner was a Notre Dame grad who had been in the Peace Corps and decided to stay in the islands after his assignment was finished.

> The Hobbit House had many promotions that were quite funny. The dwarf staff would do line dances to current popular dance songs on stage during the evening. The dwarf bouncer walked around wearing a spike collar leading a Great Dane on a leash. The dog was much larger than the hobbit. On St. Patrick's Day, the servers dressed in green like leprechauns and served green beer. They would dress like elves at Christmas. It was all done in good fun and the hobbits and customers loved it.

I had the pleasure of returning to Manila on a business trip in 2016, about thirty-five years after graduation, and the bar had become a huge tourist attraction. The Los Angeles Times wrote about The Hobbit House, claiming it was the best bar in the world. When I arrived, Jim Turner was still there and welcomed me with a big hug. I could not believe his liver was still functional. The Filipino dwarf general manager remembered me and came running over. He had been a brand-new bartender when I used to hang out there. We took some memorable photos, and I was proud to see how well they had done as owners. Jim maintained a small interest in the bar after he turned it over to the staff. One of our old friends had called ahead to tell them I was coming, and they had posted a big sign at the front door "Welcome back Mike Manyak, MD." Unfortunately, this unique bar finally closed in 2018.

Breaks from school in the Philippines took on a different tenor than back in the States. It was too far and too expensive to go home for Christmas and other holiday breaks, so we managed to have other diversions. The first Christmas I was invited to Hong Kong, one of my favorite cities, which was very exotic in those days, a true oriental-occidental mixture in a stunning setting of mountains running into the seas. Christmas in Hong Kong was very festive with many parties to attend in between tennis and side trips on a hydroplane to the city-state Macao, the gambling capital of the world. Have you ever seen a casino with hundreds of Chinese women playing mahjong? It is chaos.

We were invited to the Royal Hong Kong Club for the New Year celebration, a black-tie event for 3000 guests. The next day, our host held an "eye- opener" New Year's Day party starting about noon, still way too early because we got home at dawn. I chatted with some attorneys and then we were whisked off to another party where the VP of Mattel toy company had all the expat young kids with all kinds of toys flying through the air and careening around on the ground. We left a few hours later, hoping we could finally take it easy.

But when we returned home, the "eye-opener" party had morphed into a sundowner, and everybody was quite lively and boisterous. Our host's mother was playing old piano favorites from their era and some partiers were quite inebriated, including the general counsel, who was wearing the proverbial lampshade. Since my host knew Hong Kong, he poured the attorney into a cab with him, and I went to drive his wife in their car. I could not believe they had my absolute dream car, a 1952 MG TD British racing green convertible. She told me to drive. The driver's seat was on the right side because Hong Kong being British, vehicles drove on the left. What a thrill to drive that car on a full moonlit night through the Hong Kong mountains!

Years later, I was able to get a replica of this car, called an Allison 1952 MGTD. It was one of 750 fiberglass body exact replicas made. Except these replicas had a very strange VW three speed automatic engine. It looked exotic but could not beat a fast dog. Who cared? But you had to be careful when you took it out because it took fifteen minutes to put up the convertible top. I learned that lesson the hard way. I was invited to a late spring corporate dinner at the British embassy in Washington. I ventured out on a beautiful clear evening in the iconic British MG replica about fifteen minutes from my house. Everything was fine until in the middle of dinner when I saw a flash of lightning. The weather forecast had not predicted any rain. I ran out to the car and tried to get the top up quickly, but unsuccessfully. The heavens opened and I got soaked. I did get the top up, kind of, but had to scrunch down to see out the windshield which had a tiny wiper allowing me about six inches diameter of sight. I crawled home shivering and vowed never to be caught like that again. My kids loved the car; they were small and could ride on the wide fender in the local Fourth of July and Labor Day parades. My wife, however, hated it because it occupied her spot in the garage when I took it home. I kept it for eight years but then reluctantly sold it. It sure was a head turner though.

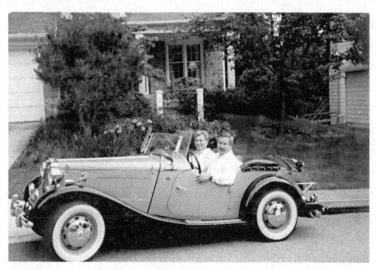

Allison MGTD replica that looked great but could not beat a fast dog. Only 750 of these were made.

I spent another Christmas during medical school in a very remote spot in the northern Philippines, in the Mountain Province. There was a youth hostel run by the Episcopalian clergy in the tiny town of Sagada with nearby waterfalls where one could swim, with interesting pagan burial grounds, and with some caves to explore. It was strikingly beautiful but quite remote and it took half a day to drive up into the mountains by private car. We didn't want to risk taking a bus on dangerous roads with precarious hairpin curves and reckless drivers which included the bus driver.

There are three words in use in English that have origins in the Philippines. One is "yo-yo" which is the name for a hunting weapon used by primitive natives who would sit in a tree and drop a rock attached to a cord onto an animal on the trail. Americans brought that weapon back to the U. S. and it evolved into a children's toy. Another word "amok" is used to describe someone who goes crazy, as in "running amok" and comes from the Malay language originally. The third is "boondocks" which means somewhere quite remote. This comes from an aberration of the name of the town Bontoc which means mountain in Tagalog and is the capital of the Mountain Province. We passed near Bontoc on our way to Sagada with spectacular terraced rice paddies way up in the mountains which is a man-made engineering marvel. That is how remote it is.

Sagada came up again a few years later when I was in residency and my boss asked me to see a patient with him who was from the Philippines. I was surprised to see a very American looking guy who I found out was a priest who had come all the way back to Washington DC for treatment. When asked where he was from in the Philippines, fully expecting Manila as the response, he said he was from the north. After ascertaining I knew a fair amount about the Philippines, he finally said he was from Sagada. He about fell out of the bed when I told him I had been there and stayed in the Episcopalian youth hostel in that tiny very remote place which he now headed.

Another memorable holiday to Hong Kong during med school occurred with Scott Harrison who was the political officer of the U.S. embassy in the Philippines. This is basically an intelligence position and Scott was CIA though he did not admit that for years. In fact, there were others who were also in the agency under cover of embassy assignments. Scott lived in the compound of the Philippine vice president right on the ocean. The VP gave Scott a list of his favorite Philippine Air Lines flight attendants to contact, a treasure map for us two single guys.

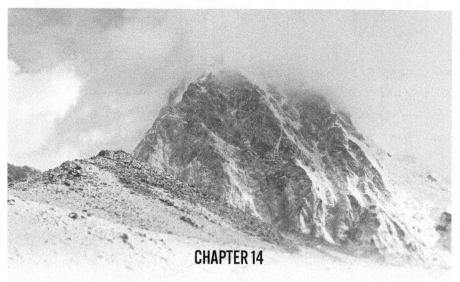

CHAPTER 14

MODELING AND MOVIES

Back at medical school in Manila the week following our dive trip with the shipwreck rescue, the local newspapers picked up the story as frontpage headline news. Two weeks later, Ma'an's TV talk show featured the story and she intended to emphasize the chronic problem of safety violations related to too many passengers and significant overload of cargo. She was furious about the blatant ignoring of safety parameters. On the segment, Maan had explained that much of the actual rescue footage had been accidentally destroyed by the contracted film developer, but she had salvaged some and would show it right after the next commercial break.

The last advertisement during the break was the Hope cigarette commercial where I appeared. Hope was the best-selling commercial brand of cigarettes in the Philippines and this ad was widely shown on television and appeared on the back covers of Time, Newsweek, and other popular magazines. If you went to the movies during that time, the ad was often shown with the upcoming attractions. It was very strange seeing my face on a big screen.

Flashing immediately to the rescue scenes, the only ones that were still viable were the images of a few of us carrying patients onto the boat to be transported to the regional hospital. So, immediately after close ups of me in the cigarette commercial hang gliding was a quick switch to a close-up clip of me carrying patients after this sea rescue. Of course, I was greeted by jeers from my friends watching this unfold while they peppered me with empty beer cans. Fame is indeed fleeting.

Many years later when I returned to the Philippines to speak at a large conference, some of the Filipinos told me that the ad campaign had run again for two years recently and was very popular. Of course, I was never notified, nor did I receive compensation. Apparently, I was a star of sorts and recently, someone found the ads on the internet and projected it on the big screen TV in a bar. My friends with me were astounded but now they knew I wasn't lying when I said that I had been in print and TV ads. Indeed, some of the grandmothers and mothers might remember me. In fact, recently at a party I met a younger Filipina lady who absolutely remembered both my popular cigarette and jeans advertisements. She was amazed and we had a good laugh.

Back in the med school days, the reason I was in the Hope cigarette commercial, one of the most widely shown throughout the country, was really a fluke. My modeling experiences were a result of a serendipitous encounter at a Manila bank at the end of my second year in medical school. I got a call from a stranger who said his friend had seen me in the bank and had recommended me as a potential model. I have to say that I didn't think this was a legitimate inquiry. I explained that I was a medical student, but I would listen to their pitch provided I could keep my clothes on during filming.

I received calls from this small agency on and off over the next several months. Frankly, it was a hassle to go to some usually distant location in the huge sprawling city of Manila with no reward for my efforts. Afterall, my purpose for being there was to attend medical school, not to pursue an acting career. Even if I scored a commercial shoot, the pay was quite low. I decided to be my own agent to avoid having the agent take a commission.

I became rather jaundiced about these calls for opportunities after nothing materialized following several calls. I decided, however, to try one last time when the agency called and told me I was perfect for an ad campaign for a fledgling jeans company. When I arrived at the ad agency, they quickly threw me a pair of jeans. But the funny thing is that the jeans they provided were intended for Filipinos who are smaller than Americans and I could not possibly squeeze into them. As we looked at each other, I told them I had my own jeans on and perhaps these could work. They agreed, so after signing a contract with them, we proceeded to the first site of the shoot which was held at an ornate five-star hotel.

In the first scene, the director instructed me to throw a jean jacket over my shoulder, and then to trot up a big marble staircase covered with a red carpet. Two very attractive female models in jeans were to walk down the stairs in the opposite direction. I was to smile at the girls, then look at their jeans as they passed, turn to the camera, and smile and say, "Wow!" before continuing up the stairs. We did a dry run which the director liked, then we filmed the scene. The photographer was quite friendly and after that scene he complimented me. "Hey Mike, you are good modeling. How long have you been doing commercials?" I told him, "This is my first one, but I've been doing THAT for ten years." He laughed as we left for other locations. It turned out he was considered the top photographer in the Philippines, and he recommended me for several commercials and to several other agencies. Although I was apprehensive about doing this, it turned out to be fun. I just had to be myself. We had a good time filming.

Following the modest success of the first jeans advertising campaign, I was contacted by a large advertising company about auditioning for an extensive ad campaign for Jag Jeans, a brand still popular today. Despite still being skeptical, I agreed but was rather dismayed when I showed up at the audition to find a large contingent of young men including local movie stars, popular athletes, and weightlifters in line to be screened. Thinking this was a huge waste of time, I still waited my turn.

The slogan for the campaign was "She wants my Jag. I will give it to her." All I could think was how inappropriate the theme appeared. When it came time for my audition shots, I told them that the theme was very weak, but they replied that the client had selected it. Then when it came to taking the shots, they wanted me to unbutton the top of my pants. I declined to do that and suggested instead that we shoot with my thumbs hooked into my belt and they agreed. After multiple poses in a sweltering, humid room where we were all sweating, I was given the standard farewell that they would get back to me. I was quite surprised when they later called and announced I had been chosen.

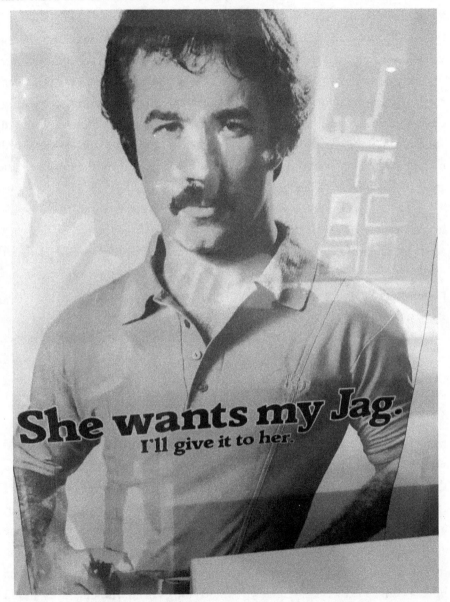

Poster advertising Jag Jeans displayed throughout the country

The follow up shoot consisted of multiple poses and several shots with different shirts. I was told to expect this in the newspaper within a few weeks. Without notification of the campaign start, early one morning I walked in to start my shift in the hospital wards to find the newspaper ad taped over the doorway to our locker area. It was nearly life-size, encompassing a full page of the Manila Bulletin, the widely read equivalent of the NY Times in this city of 20 million people. I knew this meant I was in for some serious verbal abuse. This ad ran for over three months and was in the paper three times a week. Halfway through the campaign they switched the photo to one with an additional six insets of me added along the bottom in different poses with different shirts. They made posters of this ad which were prominently displayed all over the country. I was a bit overwhelmed because I frequently was stopped on the street to sign autographs in this huge city amid comments that "There is the Jag Man."

Very soon, I was approached for a campaign for Hope cigarettes, the top-selling cigarette brand in the Philippines. The audition waiting room was filled with athletes, weightlifters, male models, and TV stars. I seriously doubted that I would be selected but I stayed there for the interview. When it was my turn, the photographer told me to turn to the left and the right as he snapped photos of me smoking without a shirt.

I did get the call back. Now I had to ask the dean for three days off to film at an offsite location outside Manila in the mountains. Getting time off from med school was not easy. You just about had to claim your mother died and you better bring back funeral flowers and a lock of her hair. Dean Fernando Sanchez, however, was a friend. He had trained at Johns Hopkins, and I aced his class on preventative medicine. He was a huge basketball fan and had attended UE games where I had played. I needed his permission to miss school for a few days. However, I was in the top 10 percent of students, and he granted my request for time off provided I made up the work missed. Med school was still my priority and he understood that.

The crew loaded up a Winnebago for the three-day shoot. I stayed in the air-conditioned trailer filled with beer, soda, and snacks awaiting filming. Filming the first shoot day, I headed to the 800-foot cliff where two champion hang-gliders hired as stunt men were sailing down towards the cameras. Although they would do the actual flying, the producer wanted to do landing shots with me. This was quite difficult because I had to jump off the end of an angled 40-foot-long ramp graduating from 3 to 8-feet in height. The problem is that the hang-gliding gear is quite bulky, and I had to run to gain momentum for the wings to operate. Imagine jumping off the runway with no control. I felt like Icarus from Greek mythology trying to fly to the sun. With significant skepticism, I donned my assigned white jumpsuit with long sleeves and long pants, and helmet with the logo, and attached the 40-foot rigid wingspan. Sweating profusely already, the bulky gear made it worse. On the signal, I ran up the ramp and jumped into space. Control was difficult because there was no air lift under the wings. The cameramen dove out of the way as I smashed to the ground in a crash landing. For their safety and mine, I was relieved that we got the closeup shots of the landing in the second take.

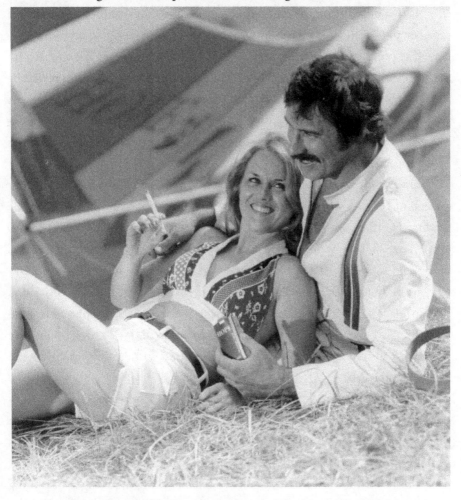

Hope cigarette commercial 1979. This was on television every night and on many top magazine covers.

The next scene engaged a blonde about my age, the wife of a counsellor in the U.S. Embassy. We snuggled up reclined on the grassy landscape and smiled at each other as she lit my cigarette for the rolling cameras. The wind kept blowing out the matches frustrating our attempts to get shots with the lighted cigarette. The producers were quite pleased as the three-day shoot concluded. Before long, the campaign for the Hope cigarette brand was running and playing everywhere.

Other whimsical opportunities arose for acting. I was cast in a very low budget movie about a bionic boy, a takeoff on a very popular TV show, *The Six Million Dollar Man*. However, *Dynamite Johnson Bionic Boy, Part Two*, was decidedly NOT a huge hit. In the Philippine version, I was the doctor who performed the operation of the body part replacements so the bionic boy could be a superhero. The props and sets were pathetic. The operating room had just a table with a white cloth. We did not wear masks. My operating utensils were a screwdriver and wrench. It was a far cry from surgical reality or even Hollywood. My only part was very short, which was fine with me. The only consolation I derived from this was that my name was in large letters on the marquee at select theaters where this movie appeared. How amusing to be on a marquee!

This was my second such experience with movies in the Philippines. Near the end of my first year in med school I was approached by an American movie producer working with Francis Ford Coppola who was filming *Apocalypse Now* in the islands. They were looking for some American extras to portray soldiers in the epic movie about the Vietnam war. I auditioned and got a one-line speaking part as a second lieutenant during a battle. It had quite a cast with Marlon Brando playing the crazy officer and Martin Sheen, Dennis Hopper, Harrison Ford, Robert Duvall, and Laurence Fishburne co-starred. However, I would have to be there all summer and would be paid very little, so I declined, preferring to get back home to see my family and friends.

I did some smaller ads, but the Jag jeans and Hope cigarettes were the mainstays for my short-lived brush as a model. After I moved out of my apartment in Manila, the two friends who rented my apartment told me later that Nike sports clothing, Gleem toothpaste, J&J baby shampoo, a nutrition drink, more clothing companies, and various other companies came knocking inquiring about hiring me to promote their products.

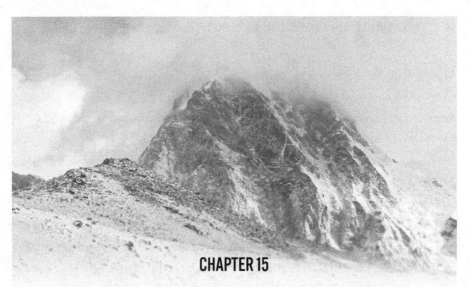

CHAPTER 15

FRIENDS FROM LETTERED AGENCIES

Another benefit of overseas living is that you meet characters from all walks of life you would not ordinarily cross paths with. Scott Harrison was a fascinating individual with very interesting insight and great sense of humor. He became one of my very closest friends for thirty-five years. He was a very experienced scuba diver who encouraged me to become scuba certified, eventually leading to the South China sea rescue. Certification was quite difficult because we had to retrieve our gear dropped at 35 feet in choppy Manila Bay. It wasn't easy but it sure gave us confidence with a real-life simulation.

Scott and I first met as the organizers of the Sunday softball league in Manila. Scott was an excellent writer with an outstanding wry sense of humor that enabled him to appreciate and survive the humorous quirks of life in the Philippines and then later Africa and China. Softball brought a bit of Americana to the Philippines for many of us ex-pats on Sunday afternoons. The Manila expat community formed eight teams and included staff from the U.S. embassy, the US Marine Corps embassy guards, American businesspeople, employees of Union Oil, the

Manila Polo Club members, medical and veterinarian school students, Peace Corps members, and the Philippines national baseball team. It was an interesting diverse cross section of lifestyles and occupations. Competition was intense while hot dogs and beer were the trademarks of league games.

Transient travelers frequently joined in when in town. So it was that no one paid much attention when Scott brought along a guy who had been doing trade negotiations at the embassy that week. The guest was short, stocky, bald, 15-pounds overweight, sweating profusely in the Philippine heat......a typical mid-50s businessman. We put him at catcher which is often the weakest or least athletic guy on the team. This time it was a little bit different. The rowdy spectators razzed us and the guy when he came up at the end of our lineup. No one had noticed he had very thick wrists. He proceeded to smack a very long, high home run which the crowd attributed to luck......until he hit another one the next time up. Now the crowd was getting a bit suspicious, but the truth did not come out until festivities after the game. Our older overweight catcher was an all-time great hitter in the baseball Hall of Fame, Harmon Killibrew, who hit 573 career home runs. We were always looking to one up the other guy and Scott sure carried that day. In later years, Scott's son summed up our attitude quite well. At that time, I was about to depart on an expedition to determine if rumors of a large unknown animal deep in the Congo was a relict dinosaur, unlikely but certainly interesting. He said very insightfully, "You know, if you ever find that dinosaur, my dad will have to find an alien." We all had a good laugh at that comment.

I did get the better of him one memorable time. In the late 1990s, Scott was notified that he was going to receive a very prestigious medal from the intelligence community to be awarded at CIA headquarters in Langley, Virginia. My wife and I were on his guest list for the ceremony which took place in front of a few hundred guests and CIA officials. At the following reception, another female CIA agent I knew in the Philippines asked if I wanted to meet the director, George Tenet. When we went to meet him, I was struck by the strong resemblance to a good friend of mine with whom I had trained early in my career in New York, Bill Tenet. When I asked him if he was related to any doctors in New York, he gave me a strange look. When I told him that Bill Tenet had been a good friend of mine during my training, he told me that Bill was his brother. We had a good laugh about him always giving George a hard time about his cholesterol level. After he left to circulate for a while, he returned from way across the large room to give me a big hug and one more laugh right in front of Scott. Scott could not believe it. "How do you know HIM??" Scott demanded to know. I found out later when I called Bill that George was his twin brother.

There were several other great stories about Scott over the years related to his career and others in which I participated. He was a CIA chief of mission in six different countries. Briefly, he was present when the body of Emperor Haile Selassie was uncovered in Ethiopia, he salvaged the Sultan of Zanzibar's flagship sunk near Dar es Salaam in 1857 (and brought me a large brass bolt which I cherish to this day), and he lived overlooking Tiananmen Square in Beijing where we observed the festivities and fireworks the night Hong Kong was returned to China from the British after 156 years of British rule in 1997. Scott reminded us that we were under 24-7 surveillance even in his apartment, so of course I had to give my wife a hard time telling her she was being watched in the shower. There were several excellent scuba dives in the spectacular waters of the South China Sea over four years including one that we descended to 220 feet on regular oxygen, not tri-mix gases. While that is not advisable for safety reasons, Scott wanted to practice decompression stops for emergencies and felt I was accomplished enough to accompany him on this spectacular wall dive with different fish and sharks at different levels. However, I vowed not to do that again.

Ric Jacobson is another longtime friend and former CIA station chief in several countries. He and Scott served together in Vietnam and spent time in Laos where the US officially was not present. John Mercer was a CIA agent friend stationed at the embassy in Manila and whom we were able to catch up with later in Washington. We all had common ground living in Manila, and it was great fun to get back together. John Mercer was in the news again in the early 2000s when the Taliban overran Afghanistan and jailed his Christian missionary daughter Heather. John went on the international news media offering himself in exchange for his daughter's release, a probable death sentence given his CIA background. Fortunately, she was rescued by special forces who raided the jail and freed her from that hellhole in a chaotic scene. I heard some crazy stories over the years from these guys. One of my favorites was told to me by Ric one night at our favorite DC hangout, the Prime Rib. The story concerned the saga of the supposed enormous deposit strike at Busang, East Kalimantan, by Bre-X Corporation mining engineer David Walsh and his geologist Filipino partner Michael de Guzman. The American mining conglomerate Freeport-McMoRan, was a prospective partner in developing the site. This discovery by Canadian-based Bre-X Minerals skyrocketed their stock price from a penny stock to nearly $300 a share.

The fraud began to unravel rapidly in March, 1997, when de Guzman reportedly committed suicide by jumping from a plane in Indonesia. Ric was the intelligence agent sent to investigate. A body was found four days later in the jungle, with surgically-removed missing hands and feet. In addition, the body was reportedly mostly eaten by animals. Ric evaluated the body and told me the abdomen had a long incision that was stitched up. According to journalist John McBeth, a body had gone missing from the morgue of the town from which the helicopter flew. The remains of "de Guzman" were found only 400 meters from a logging road. No one saw the body except another Filipino geologist who claimed it was de Guzman. One of the five women who considered themselves his wife was receiving monetary payments from somebody long after the supposed death of de Guzman. Bre-X collapsed in 1997 and its shares became worthless in one of the biggest stock scandals in Canadian history, and the biggest mining scandal of all time after the gold samples were found to be fraudulent.

This whole story was the subject of the movie *Gold* starring Matthew McConaughey. Michael de Guzman supposedly escaped to the Philippines, something that does not shock me.

Scott and Ric had a humorous running battle trying to outdo the other. I remember when Scott transferred to Tanzania as CIA station chief, he would send Ric postcards of topless African women with unequal breasts to the Manila embassy addressed to Ric from his girlfriend. Of course, I would get some mailed to me as well. What was so irritating to Ric was that they went through the embassy mailroom, and everyone saw them and got a good laugh. Ric finally got even with Scott when he went down to the Hobbit House and rounded up the full dwarf staff for a photo of them lined up from the shortest to the tallest. He had them smiling at the camera and facing sideways in a line with a hand on the shoulder of the dwarf in front. Ric made this into a postcard and sent it with the following message, "Dear Dad, when are you coming home? We all miss you. Everyone says we look like you". This, of course, went through the embassy mail room in Dar es Salaam where everyone could see it. I think Scott stopped sending Ric those postcards. Dwarf jokes may not be politically correct nowadays, but it was hilarious nonetheless and the hobbits loved it, they knew Bwana Scott well.

Scott had a wicked sense of humor that I loved. When he was in the Philippines, he organized a rally at the Russian embassy on the first anniversary of the Russians being kicked out of Afghanistan. He arranged with a Filipino big business magnate friend Freddy Elizalde to get 5000 of his employees to go to the Russian embassy with a promise of free hot dogs and apple pie. What is more American than hot dogs and apple pie? And Filipinos like nothing more than a party and free food. They misread the significance of such an event and thought it was a true celebration. What a finger in the eye of the Russians! Scott told me later he saw his Russian intelligence counterpart at a good restaurant a day or so later and the Russian just vigorously extended his middle finger repeatedly. These spooks were all declared intelligence guys and of course knew each other and had to interact in diplomatic circles. That image still makes me chuckle.

> Scott transferred to Tanzania, and he loved being called Bwana (meaning mister in KiSwahili) because it reminded him of the Tarzan movies, we all saw as kids. In the Tarzan movies, Tarzan would yell "Ungowa!" and the charging elephants would come to a screeching halt. But Bwana Scott learned that it actually meant "entangled" so it made no sense when Tarzan used it. When Scott would get on a rant, I would say "Ungowa Bwana" loudly to him and it always elicited big laughs.

Scott was a prolific writer with a wry sense of humor for the ironies of life, especially in the foreign outposts where he was assigned. I still have a box of his letters with many anecdotes, these should have been published. Receiving a letter from Scott always perked me up even in the midst of my eighty-to-one-hundred-hour internship hours which was like being Ben Hur in the slave galley pulling an oar, especially compared to the life I had in Manila. Scott had begged me to come back to Manila for a visit and said he would have his multi-billionaire friend Freddy Elizalde's dark green Rolls limo filled with hobbits and Miss Philippines meet me on the tarmac. No one gets to do that in the Marcos era of martial law, but Scott and Freddy could. I really could not get the time off so had to pass on what I am sure would have been a most entertaining vacation.

Another letter arrived from Scott one day that really made my week. I had become very enamored of a beautiful Filipina magazine cover model. She worked in marketing for the Hotel Intercontinental and we hung out with several such friends there. Unfortunately, she had an American boyfriend who was the general manager of the five-star Philippine Plaza Hotel. I gave it the old college try but could not wrest her away, which was too bad. After I left Manila, Scott told me the boyfriend was transferred to the Athens Plaza Hotel and she had gone with him. Scott had been passing through Athens and learned she was there. What does he do? He sent her a dozen roses from me saying how much I missed her. My wingman, watching out for me! He figured she would be looking behind every potted plant for me.

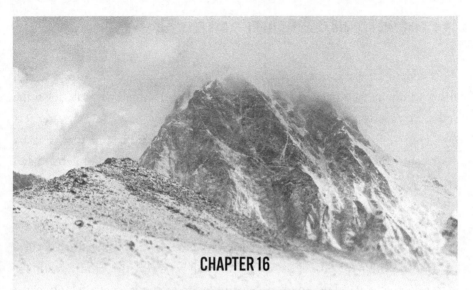

CHAPTER 16

THE BAMBOO PALACE
AND SPANISH TREASURE

s I mentioned, one of Scott's close friends was Freddie Elizalde, arguably the second most powerful man in the Philippines after President Marcos. Freddie was a multi-billionaire who owned very large corporations ranging from the long-distance telephone concession to the national electric company. He was a Spanish Filipino with blonde hair and blue eyes and was a former Olympic swimmer for the Philippines who also dabbled as a sculptor. Freddie had multiple large houses in different provinces and frequently held parties in his nearby palatial mountain retreat. He would send his Winnebago, tricked out in white shag carpeting and huge sound system, to pick us up for parties. But you never know whether your companions will be South American countesses or foreign diplomats. When we arrived for his wife's birthday party with two hundred guests, we were milling about with drinks and food when an argument broke out upstairs on the circular balustrade.

Suddenly, firearms appeared and one guy with an automatic weapon started firing wildly in the direction of the crowd as a victim fell all the way down the stairs. Everybody screamed and dove under tables, me included. Only after several tense minutes did we realize Freddie had hired a stunt troupe to simulate a very realistic home invasion. We laughed uneasily as we dusted ourselves off and resumed partying. Scott told me another time a few hundred elegantly dressed guests had to trudge through mud to a banquet hall before being served a specialty known as Chinese Soup #5. This soup is a broth with bull genitals cut into small pieces and is said to be an aphrodisiac. Freddie however had all waiters remove the soup tureen covers with a flourish to reveal the broth…with the intact bull genitalia in the soup. Because of Freddie's status, guests felt obligated to eat the soup. You had to be on your toes at his parties because he loved to surprise people.

Freddie had a very unusual three-story bamboo palace on the beach on the island of Boracay, rightfully renowned as one of the most beautiful beaches in the world. Spectacularly stunning multi-hued blue green waters are framed by a mile or so of pristine fine white sand the texture of baby powder. Boracay has now become a tourist destination and overcrowded but then it was bucolic, with offshore coral reefs and shipwrecks with diverse marine life. Freddie's three-story Bamboo Palace was unique with its stunning views. The province of Aklan where Boracay is located is the home to the Philippine equivalent of Carnival complete with big parade floats, masks, and colorful costumes.

Freddie re-entered my life years later after I had dived to the famous treasure galleon *Senora Nuestra de Atocha* in the Florida Keys. The *Atocha* was part of the Spanish treasure fleet that sank after hitting a reef in a hurricane in 1622 on its way to Spain with 264 lives lost. A second hurricane followed shortly after the one that sank the *Atocha*, scattering salvagers and the remainder of the ship down the reef. Pat Clyne was the photographer on the day of discovery in 1985 by Mel Fisher's treasure hunters. My favorite night on the ship at the *Titanic* site was when Pat regaled us with a three-hour description of finding the *Atocha*. His tale of bringing up cannons and long gold chains was entrancing. Pat invited me to dive the treasure trail because they were still finding treasure and artifacts every year. Who could resist that?

On our dives we recovered artifacts like pieces- of-eight Spanish silver coins and a spectacular 24-carat finely filigreed gold piece from the princess of Spain's belt. We were told that we could keep any emerald we found worth up to $40,000. We did not delay getting into the water.

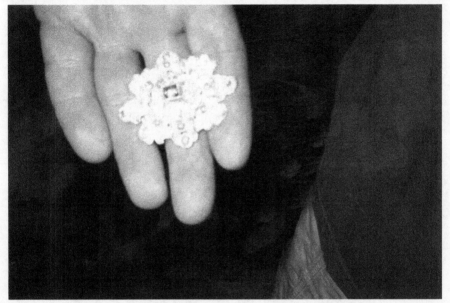

The 24-carat beautifully filigreed piece of the Princess of Spain found on our dive trip on the treasure galleon *Senora Nuestra de Atocha.*

I spent time with the curators of their finds in the lab at their Key West Museum. Holding old cutlasses and flaring old muskets called arquebuses conjured up dreams of conquistadors. Likewise, for seeing and holding serious treasure. My wife came down for festivities hosted by the museum and we were invited into the vault where Kim Fisher, Mel's son, and the corporate president, told her to hold out her hands. He draped 20 feet of heavy gold chains around her shoulders and placed a huge emerald in each hand. The emeralds were roughly 30 carats worth about $3 million each and of the highest quality from the Colombian mines the Spanish had looted.

Talk about wrecks of treasure ships led to a discussion about potential salvage in the Philippine waters where it was known that 19 Spanish treasure galleons had gone down in the 17th and 18th centuries. Pat outlined how we could mount an expedition to search for these treasure wrecks with proper financial backing.

He shared with me a map of the known sites. Scott Harrison and I approached Freddie to see if he would finance such a venture. We flew to Manila when I was on a business trip in Asia. Scott at that time lived in Hong Kong and Manila after he retired from the CIA and ran his own security agency. When we laid this all out to Freddie, our question in addition to funding was whether the notoriously corrupt police and military would allow us to keep (or share) any artifacts that we retrieved. Since this venture would cost approximately one million dollars, it was imperative that what we recovered could be kept. After much serious discussion with Freddie, he concluded that if we found anything, the government would confiscate it. Even with his pull we would not be protected. What a shame to have to pass on this incredible opportunity. Here I still sit with a bona fide treasure map and cannot search for the treasure with any degree of safety or confidence that we could keep what we recovered.

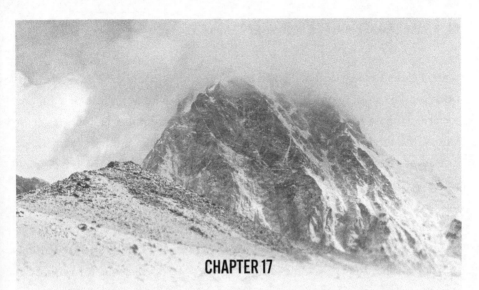

CHAPTER 17

RESIDENCY TRAINING IN THE BIG APPLE

We were delayed leaving the Philippines after graduation because of a typhoon as well as mundane chores like selling the Mercedes, shipping items, purchasing last minute presents, and making endless rounds of farewell parties. Some of us dragged our feet and I was reticent to leave this good life. I was on television every night, had many good friends whom I might not see again, scuba diving on the weekends, and other activities. Leaving my pet monkey was not easy and I left Juju with a good family. I spent my last night before leaving Manila in a five-star hotel with several friends overlooking Manila Bay during one more typhoon.

Medical degree in hand, I now had to undergo several years of specialty training. After a month's stay in Michigan, I moved to New York City to begin my postgraduate training at Booth Memorial Medical Center, a program affiliated with New York University School of Medicine. I remained at Booth as a general surgery resident for three years. Booth was a busy Level One trauma center with a very active clinical staff in all disciplines except pediatrics. During my time there, I gained a great deal of clinical experience in patient management. We routinely worked close to one hundred hours a week, leaving very little time for any social activities. (Today, there are hospital limits on the number of hours residents work.) The three years in general surgery clarified my desire to be a subspecialist instead of a general surgeon. At that time CT scans were new, and the hospital rule was that a physician had to be present when the intravenous contrast was injected in case there was an allergic reaction. It would be a poor use of resources to have a highly paid radiologist present, so the department used residents to inject the contrast. I got wind of that opportunity and was good friends with the radiology techs. They placed me on the call schedule for residents. If I worked for a week while I was already in the hospital, I could make about $1000 per week. I told the techs to call me if they couldn't reach the resident on call. They did. I ended up making several hundred dollars a week and no longer had to moonlight in off hours at another hospital.

With little time for recreation, we did manage to attend baseball games at Shea stadium, the home of the New York Mets. It was cheap entertainment and Shea stadium was close to the hospital. Unbelievably, two games in a row I caught a foul ball baseball souvenir. After the second one, I got a tap on the shoulder and the women behind me asked if they could get a photo. One of them, Randye Ringler, was the group sales manager for the Mets and they wanted that for a marketing photo. She ended up giving me a press pass for helping her market a Booth Memorial Hospital Night at the stadium which allowed me to go to games free.

A few years later, back in Washington, Randye called and offered me box seats for the World Series because I was a Mets fan when they were lousy and so deserved tickets for loyalty when they were very good. I was only able to get to one game but went to the same side gate from years before, only now it was mobbed but the same security guard was there and remembered me. As I turned from him and went in, I literally bumped right into model Christie Brinkley who said, "Hi, how are you?" thinking she knew me. I responded, "Great, how are you? Where are we going after the game?". She said she was not sure, but we should catch up and meet back here. My friend was completely speechless.

Our box seats included the trainer for the *Karate Kid* movie protagonist Ralph Macchio, who also joined us. We saw one of the iconic great World Series games.

We were in first base box seats when late in the game, a famous error was made allowing the Mets to win the game. That play is a highlight shown nearly every year at World Series time. Afterward, Randye took me down into the dugout area where we chatted with some Mets as Howard Johnson, who had hit forty-seven home runs that year, came down in his briefs and a full-length mink coat. Sadly, I never caught up with Christie Brinkley.

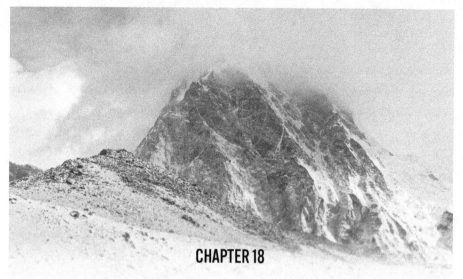

CHAPTER 18

CRUISING THE CARIBBEAN

The only respite during residency while in New York came when I had an incredible opportunity to be the ship doctor on a cruise liner for Norwegian Caribbean Lines (NCL) in 1982. I was sharing stories about the Philippines when on call at the emergency room in the early morning with the chairman of the department. His close friend was the medical director of NCL, and the department chair volunteered to call him on my behalf to see if I could get on the schedule. The only obstacle was that I had to work a minimum of one month and that was all that I had for personal time off for the year. The program did not allow you to take it all at once, but I was able to cajole our program manager because of this unique possibility.

So, I headed to Miami to be on the *MS Sunward*, the smallest of the NCL fleet at 850 feet. These were shorter cruises for a few days from Miami to Freeport and Nassau in the Bahamas, then for to a private island for a big barbecue, then back to Miami. I would have an afternoon in Miami to get off the ship and then board again for the next cruise. At first, I was upset because I wanted one of the larger ships with longer cruises, but it turns out that the shorter cruise was cheaper. This had two benefits. First, it was cheaper so that it meant that younger people could afford to cruise and the capacity was less than the larger ships. These shorter cruises were like one big party. Second, because this younger population was on the ship less time on than other cruises and was much healthier, the medical personnel had a more relaxed time with fewer expected emergencies.

I met with the captain and the executive officer. As the ship physician, I needed to be in the clinic one hour in the morning in uniform and one hour in the afternoon in bathing suit and shirt, then be on call. The fulltime ICU nurse who was my assistant had been on the ship for eight years and was very experienced. As the physician, I was the third ranking officer, and the ship could not leave port without me on board per maritime law. They issued me a white officer's uniform with gold-striped epaulettes. I was also given an electronic pager for short messages.

This was a good deal for me. In addition to a king size suite with daily laundry service and all meals, I had a free bar tab, so I was able to order champagne for selected guests. This was not a bad part-time job for a poor resident.

If a passenger needed attention outside of the brief clinic hours, the person would contact the bell captain who could handle most non-emergencies. If more medical knowledge was required, the nurse would be contacted before I was alerted. There was a small infirmary in the clinical space where we could evaluate and treat someone.

It was important to establish a protocol to respond to an emergency, because communication is key in these situations. Meeting with the captain clarified this issue. If I felt we needed to evacuate a passenger or crew member, I would make the medical decision. It would then be up to the captain to manage the logistics of the evacuation.

Although we had a few cases where more sophisticated medical care was required, we only had one incident requiring evacuation during my tenure. I received a call that a patient was seizing and was in the infirmary unit. When I arrived there, a relatively small guy was throwing two large Jamaican assistants all over the room. They had just subdued him, and the nurse got an IV into him and injected Valium. We added antiseizure medication. He was a crew member from the islands, and no one knew him. We didn't know if he had hit his head and had significant internal trauma, had ingested or smoked something psychogenic, had epilepsy, or had a reaction to medicine. He needed evacuation.

I ran up to the officer's mess to get something to eat while he was stable since we were now going to be busy controlling him until evacuation. The captain decided to return to Miami as the most efficient route. The ship made a very noticeable 180-degree turn, and the captain announced there was a very sick patient and that we were returning to Miami. Since all the people in the dining area could see us in the officers mess, all eyes turned toward me as I was shoveling food into my mouth. I had to stand up and wave to the passengers that the patient was stable now with a big smile.

When we landed in port, instead of a single ambulance, we were met by seven ambulances all lit up like Christmas lights. It looked like a major disaster. The man was evacuated successfully though I was told later that all tests were negative. He probably had an unrecognized epileptic focus. Another crew member also had to be evacuated. He had pain in his abdominal right lower quadrant which can be a red flag for appendicitis. He saw my predecessor two weeks earlier and had been given some antibiotics inappropriately for an unknown infection, but no other concern was raised. I could palpate a mass and suspected a peri-appendiceal abscess which is a surgical issue. Basically, this was a burst appendix walled off from spreading by the body's defenses. I called the medical director of the company to explain why I was concerned, and we agreed to get the man off at the next port. When he got to the hospital, the CT scan confirmed my diagnosis, and the man needed emergency surgery.

The crew had a half day off between cruises to go to the bank or run errands. The captain asked me to stick around on one of these breaks my second week. He had news of a problem on the MS Norway, the largest NCL cruise ship at the time with 2500 passengers. He asked me to stand by in case I was needed on that ship. The ship was incapacitated by a fire on board. The ship finally limped into a port with all the crew and passengers intact we heard later and we were able to stand down.

The ship was going to have to be transported to Bremen, Germany for repairs. NCL needed a skeleton crew to cruise to Europe and asked if I wanted to be the doctor. This was a fully paid European vacation. Unfortunately, I had to pass because I had to be back at the hospital in two weeks.

Six months after my cruise line physician position ended, I began my urology residency from 1982 to 1985 at The George Washington University Medical Center (GWU) in the heart of Washington, D.C. literally next to the White House. After my residency, this would be my professional home for the next nineteen years except for a three-year hiatus spent at the National Cancer Institute (NCI) as a fellow. GWU was in a busy traffic circle and very close to many famous and infamous landmarks and offered unique opportunities in government areas and non-profit organizations.

Early that first year, I was at a favorite DC watering hole across from GWU Medical Center. A waitress friend was talking about her vacation and how her ship caught on fire. She said they were stuck five days at sea with no air conditioning, had to ration food and water, and had to stay in their rooms. They were given a free cruise when they returned to shore to try NCL again, but she was reluctant to cruise after that harrowing experience. I asked her if she was on the *Norway*, and she confirmed.

Another chance conversation gave me more insights into how truly remarkable and horrific the ship fire could have been. A year later, as a second-year urology resident at GWU, I was moonlighting in Scranton, Pennsylvania one weekend every six weeks. It paid well. It was a four-hour drive, but after the long hours, I would be too tired to drive safely, so I took puddle jumper flights back to D.C. I stopped in Philadelphia for a connecting flight and grabbed a drink at the airport bar. I sat next to a fireman with the Coast Guard. We chatted and quickly connected some dots and found that he worked at the harbor from which naval vessels had been dispatched to fight the fire on the NCL ship.

The fireman said, "I was called to the fire on the NCL ship. It was a maritime disaster. The fire melted the steel girder beams in the engine room close to the fuel source. That fire was less than a half inch from igniting the fuel supply, which would have been a real tragedy. Thankfully we were able to put out the fire."

I had heard three different perspectives of this same story, from my captain of my ship, the passenger, and now the fireman. Thankfully the issue got resolved and the passengers were safe. This experience added to my knowledge base for planning for the unexpected in expedition medicine.

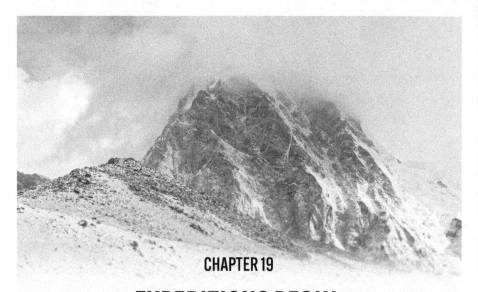

CHAPTER 19

EXPEDITIONS BEGIN: SOUTH ASIAN ADVENTURES

I n 1985 I was selected as one of four American Urological Association Scholars, the first one to secure an AUA scholarship to the National Cancer Institute (NCI). My fellowship, from 1985 to 1988, was in an esoteric field called photodynamic therapy (PDT) which consisted of administering a photosensitizing drug which concentrated initially in all tissues but then was retained in tumors for a variable time later. This created a temporary gradient between normal and abnormal tissue. When tissue was exposed to specific light wavelengths that were absorbed by that specific photosensitizing drug, abnormal tissue was selectively destroyed, and normal tissue was unaffected. The light source was produced by a laser which provides very specific light to activate the drug. This whole concept was quite intriguing because it spared normal tissue adjacent to tumor. It worked. When I moved on to GWU, I created a program with the NCI to treat superficial aggressive bladder cancer.

The results of this program culminated in the largest published series for treatment of this type of tumor with PDT. I was asked to present these and other data related to PDT and our research all over the world. This gave me an interesting niche in the academic world and a multitude of opportunities for travel.

Another phase of my life began in 1988, in addition to my urology practice. I had married at the end of my fellowship; Rebecca, my wife, was a southerner from Louisville, Kentucky, who worked as an ICU/recovery room nurse at GWU. We had three children and busy professional and personal lives. She understood the pressures and obligations I had as a surgeon and teacher and, as the children grew, she took a hiatus from nursing. My days began early in the morning and would not end until into the evening. I was home as much as I could, but my wife took on the bulk of parenting. This was really driven home to me when my kids would be asked if they were going to be doctors or nurses. My oldest daughter Rachel's response, when she was about six was, "No way, my dad is never home!"

That was an arrow to the heart for sure. I vowed to always try to spend quality time with them. I was fortunate to go on many expeditions, but it was always rewarding to get back home to my family. My only regret about any of these activities was the time away from the family. I told my son Tim, my youngest, one evening as we were watching the sky for shooting stars on our upper deck that whenever I was away, I was thinking about them and my wife. I showed Tim how to find the North Star by finding the Big Dipper and told Tim that wherever I was in the world, even in the most remote jungle or desert, that he could look up at the North Star and I would be doing the same. That way we would stay connected. He remembers that to this day.

As the children got older, I promised to take each of them individually on some form of remote expedition. Occasionally, I would ask my wife, "Do you want to go with me to Mongolia and ride camels?" or some similar activity. Invariably, the answer was, "Are you crazy? I want to explore Paris!" We certainly did some of that as well; she was not excited about most of the more exotic trips unless it involved staying at the Ritz. I have to say, she probably made the right decision on most of these. Although she could do it, I know she wouldn't have enjoyed fighting off motion sickness on the high rolling waves in the North Atlantic at the Titanic site.

> I would try to go on one expedition a year and use part of my vacation time. Most remote expeditions took three weeks at most, which was about the maximum time I could be away with my responsibilities at home.

My wife Rebecca did go on occasional trips with me. Five years into our marriage in 1993, she accompanied me to India when I was asked to join a small cadre of internationally famous urologists to give lectures in northern India. After our academic activities, we went to the well-known game reserve Kaziranga in the northeastern Indian state Assam. Assam was hard to get into for tourists because of ongoing political unrest but our hosts cleared the path for us. Kaziranga is the premier home of the Asian rhino, the one with the armored plates. During this visit, I went off with another urologist to view elephants with several guides. We got out of the jeep and walked twenty-five meters to observe an elephant herd on the other side of a small river. As we turned to go back to the jeep, the guide yelled, "Leopard! Leopard! Get in the jeep quickly!" However, the animal in the road thirty meters away watching us with crossed paws had no spots. It was a Royal Bengal tiger, a magnificent and beautiful animal. I yelled, "That is a tiger! Let's get closer!" Well, the Keystone Kops that we had as guides not only could not identify the correct animal but they also flooded the jeep so it would not start. By the time they got the jeep started, the tiger had padded off into the tall grass. Although I never did get a photo, that image is imprinted in my mind along with the thought that he knew we were there and could have attacked us at any time.

We also journeyed up into Bhutan, a very idyllic and pristine country in the Himalayan mountains. Bhutan only lets in a limited number of tourists, about 3,000 a year at that time. While we were in Bhutan we had a dinner with the Bhutanese Minister of Education, the Minister of Health, and the Minister of Foreign Affairs. Bhutanese food is a combination of Asian and western influenced dishes, heavy on the beef or yak in this case, liberally sprinkled with hot chilis and covered with a creamy cheese sauce which was usually yak cheese.

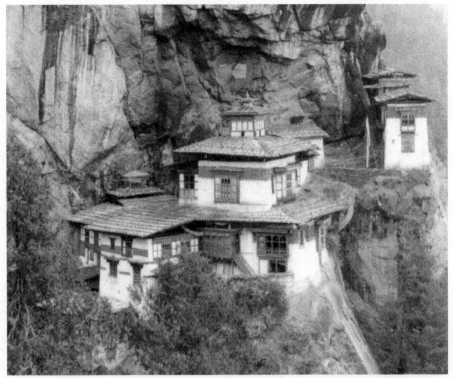

Taktsang, the 1692 Tiger's Nest Buddhist monastery in Bhutan over 10,000 feet to which we hiked.

The Tiger's Lair monastery Taktsang, a spectacular but treacherous cliffside climb nested at 10,000 feet with no rails along the ancient rocky stairway. We also toured the only hospital in the capital Thimphu. There were forty patients in the hospital, all in one ward. We made rounds and stopped to talk to one man with a horribly disfigured face. We were told he was a victim of a Himalayan bear attack. Apparently, the bears come out of hibernation in spring and farmers bending over in their fields present a good target. The head surgeon, a British educated Burmese, told me he reported on twenty-six such patients in a series at a major Asian medical meeting recently. Who else has a series of twenty-six bear attack cases? In a follow up to this story, several years later in my clinic I had a Burmese diplomat in for an examination and when I told him I had been near Burma (now Myanmar) in Bhutan, he told me his brother was a surgeon in Thimphu. He was astounded when we compared notes and found out that his brother was the same surgeon whom I had talked to in the Thimphu hospital! Once again, the medical world seemed very small.

We left Bhutan on the national airline Druk Air or Dragon Air. The airline had three planes and a very short runway exiting over spectacular Himalayan visage. I loved telling my small kids that I had flown on a dragon.

While on the road in India, we stopped in one smaller town renowned for a huge statue of a bull. Tradition had it that if someone walked around the bull three times, the person would be granted a wish. I saw my wife walking around the bull but she refused to tell me what she wished for. Several months later, back in Washington, we found out she was pregnant with our third child. Our son Tim was born and then my wife revealed she had wished for a son. We tell Tim he is part Indian. It might explain his fondness for curry and his comical Indian imitation accent. "Veddy good suh."

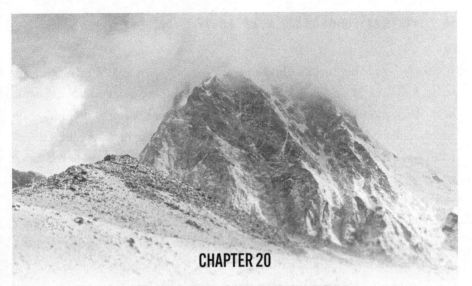

CHAPTER 20

THE NEXT GENERATION: ALASKA TO ANTARCTICA

All my children are fluent in Spanish; they attended a Spanish immersion school where we lived in the Washington suburb of Chevy Chase, Maryland. When Rachel turned fifteen, I was in southern California for business and out for dinner with long time close Notre Dame classmate Peter Burke. I told him my idea to take one of the kids at a time on a trip. His children were the same ages as mine and his daughter had some Spanish in school. He thought it would be a great idea to join us for a trip to a Spanish speaking country.

We went to Madrid, where I had been several times and loved the country. The first night there, we went to a restaurant where all the waiters and waitresses are from the Spanish opera. They wandered through the crowd pouring water or delivering cutlery and then would sit down at the table and start singing. Despite Rachel's reluctance, we went to the Prado, my favorite museum, which she loved.

Rachel made her presence known one day when we were in a taxi, and I was trying to talk to the driver. I know some basic Spanish but suddenly, Rachel sat up in the back and went off on the taxi driver in very rapid Spanish and his eyeballs were bulging as big as saucers. She then said, "Dad, stop trying to speak Spanish." I said, "Why? He understands me." She retorted, "Well, did you understand that he called you a dumb s** t?" Obviously not. Rachel told me she set him straight and told him not to disrespect her father or he would have to answer to her. Here is this young pretty blonde, obviously American, raining hellfire on him in rapid perfectly accented Spanish. She passed her real-life Spanish speaking experience with flying colors. We still laugh about this. We loved that Spanish trip!

A year or so later, son Tim jumped the queue when I was a member of the scientific advisory board (SAB) for a medical device company which had its annual SAB meeting in Alaska at a salmon fish camp. I took Tim to the camp off the coast of Ketchikan. The fish camp was a very comfortable lodge built on a two-story commercial container slightly offshore to keep the bears away. There were bears all over the place along with bald eagles. We went out in 20-foot small motorboats several times a day, so there were two of us and my twelve-year-old Tim. We caught a lot of fish, some almost bigger than him, and he enjoyed himself. The only time he got a bit agitated was when I landed a good-sized halibut which filled most of the boat as it flopped all over the place. One day he decided to go on a boat with guides looking for bears which was quite successful for him. However, that was the day I heard a "whoooosh" right behind us in our small boat with another fisherman as two 40-foot whales rose thirty feet away from us obviously checking us out.

Next, it was my middle daughter Susanna's turn in 2004. When I talked to her about where she wanted to go to use her Spanish, she did not even hesitate when she told me, "Dad, I want to go to New York City!" I laughed and said maybe that would qualify but we would do that next spring, it was December. A day or so later, I received a call from Geoff Green, owner of an award-winning educational adventure travel program "Students On Ice" where students went to the Arctic, Antarctic, and Everest. The program needed a doctor for its upcoming two-week Antarctic trip on an icebreaker, the *MV Polar Star*. I told him I would do it if I could bring one of my children. It turns out Susanna was exactly the right age for the student group accompanying the scientists to assist with their research. Geoff said she could go for half price. I called Susanna and said, "Hey Susanna, I figured out where we are going for our trip."

"Where Dad?" "We are going to the South Pole!" I replied. She exclaimed, "WHAT??!! I am not going to the South Pole!" I told her I would give her an hour to consider it, but I needed to decide right away. When I called an hour later, she said, "My friends all said that is so cool! I am definitely going!"

The group rendezvoused in Buenos Aires, Argentina, for a few days so Susanna did get to use her Spanish. Then, we flew to Ushuaia in Tierra del Fuego, Argentina, the southernmost city in the world, a beautiful place that reminded me of British Columbia with snow-topped mountains by the sea. We boarded the *MV Polar Star*, then departed for Antarctica, crossing some of the roughest seas in the world, the Drake Passage. When I gave a lecture on that segment, I was wedged between the podium and the wall, hanging on precariously with the pitching of the ship. Half of the audience was somnolent with the Dramamine they had taken for motion sickness. I remarked that I had been accused of putting the audience to sleep before but not to this extent.

You cannot imagine the natural beauty of this area with constantly shifting patterns of gray, blue, and white that are anything but monotonous. Cruising slowly past icebergs impresses one with the magnitude of the *Titanic* disaster. Amazingly, approximately 70 percent of the world's biomass lives in the Southern Ocean. There are trillions of tons of krill which are consumed by a myriad of birds and fish. The estimated 35 million seals in the area follow the fish, and the large predatory seals follow both. At the top of the food chain are the mighty and spectacular orcas.

The penguins were fascinating, and these highly inquisitive birds waddled up to us when we stopped at an island with 250,000 breeding pairs. The rule is you cannot approach them, but you can let them approach you, and believe me, they do, checking you out from head to toe. The parade of penguins marching toward you and back again looked like people on the streets of Manhattan on a busy spring day.

We had warned everyone to keep their hands out of the doorway while the ship was in rough water because the doors could suddenly slam and injure them.

Of course, Susanna was talking to me one night and I yelled to get her hand out of the doorway, but I was too late. The door slammed on her finger, and I was heartbroken. She was quite brave despite being in great pain, we immediately iced down the finger, and my examination suggested there was no fracture though x-rays would be needed to confirm that. The finger swelled significantly, and I was afraid I would have to surgically incise the finger to relieve the pressure and avoid nerve damage. Fortunately, we were able to defer that with conservative management and pain medication. I splinted the finger, and she was able to join in all activities. Although I had a couple of diabetics and asthmatics among our passengers, Susanna ended up being my most serious case.

We had to share rooms and my roommate turned out to be a most interesting and very entertaining fellow. Bill Lishman was a pioneer with ultralight aircraft and was the protagonist in the well-known movie *Fly Away Home* which depicted his efforts to re-establish migratory patterns for Canadian geese. Bill was a Canadian sculptor, filmmaker, inventor, naturalist and public speaker, described by the newspaper as a "dyslexic, colour-blind, wildly creative sculptor" whose pieces had previously been displayed at the World's Fair. We had a great time together and he filmed one of the most interesting events on the trip: adult orcas teaching their juveniles how to hunt seals by washing them off ice floes right in front of us. The staff told me they had only seen this behavior once before in the past ten years from quite a distance.

After the trip, I gladly sponsored Bill Lishman for The Explorers Club membership. The NYC-based national club is a prestigious elite professional society interested in scientific study and field exploration. A year later, I was in Toronto, and he took me to his house forty miles north of Toronto, famous throughout Canada because it was built on a 110-acre property into the hillside like one of the hobbit's houses in *The Lord of The Rings* movie. His roof was a meadow with skylights to let light into his abode. It was a unique and amazing place that was quite bright and very cozy. Bill had built an ultralight runway in front of his house to fly his seven different ultralight aircraft. He turned to me and said, "Let's go flying!"

He took me to his hangar and selected an aircraft that looked like a broomstick with a motor, which reminded me of the flying brooms in the quidditch game in the Harry Potter series. I asked where I put my feet and he pointed to a small transverse bar but then he said I could not shift my weight because that is how they steer this broomstick. The same was true for the crosspiece I was to hang onto, which also steered this vehicle. I was not amused. Fortunately, it was too windy that day, so we took out an enclosed ultralight which was so light we easily wheeled it out of the hangar ourselves. I went up in that tiny aircraft and got blown around but fortunately, did not lose my lunch.

Meanwhile, most of the adolescents on this Antarctica trip belonged to a student ambassador organization called People 2 People. Their leaders all loved Susanna and wanted her to join. She proceeded to do that after we returned and was ecstatic that the next year's trip was to Australia. Susanna reasoned correctly that her dad would not say no. She went on a fantastic three-week trip to Australia where she swam with dolphins near Cairns, sheared sheep on a farm in Queensland, and walked over the iconic bridge in Sydney Harbor. Susanna had already been to Spain on a school trip so now she had been on five continents including the most remote in Australia and Antarctica before she was sixteen-years old.

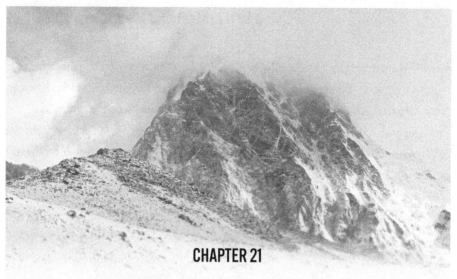

CHAPTER 21

BOMBS TO BLIZZARDS

My professional career was anything but routine. Clinical practice was varied and challenging. I shared a house with the GW VP of Medical Affairs, a colorful character. He was the youngest hospital administrator in the country at age twenty-eight. Mike Barch is a very bright individual with an extraordinary business sense with innovative ideas. While at the helm of the hospital, he revamped the hospital cafeteria and offered soft shell crabs at a great price on Fridays. This was such a good deal that the local neighbors would line up for lunch at the hospital cafeteria, something I have never seen, particularly given the usual quality of hospital food. He also instituted a gourmet ice cream kiosk in a corner of the cafeteria. His attitude and approach made GW a very vibrant place with lots of young professionals. His leadership was a major reason I came back to GW to begin my academic career. He had a vision that was contagious.

As the VP of Medical Affairs and GW Hospital Administrator, Mike was constantly being served legal papers for the continuous parade of lawsuits directed at the hospital. Most of these were frivolous but all lawsuits needed a response.

To be officially served for a lawsuit, process servers had to physically deliver the papers to the defendant and Mike, as administrator, was named on all of them. Although this process sounds relatively straightforward, he created a firewall so it could not be done easily. His office staff was instructed to never let process servers into the office and the process servers would be told he was not there. Mike had a surreptitious back door to escape. It became a game to avoid process servers. They were wily, however, and he had to be on his toes to elude them.

One late afternoon, I did not have my car and caught a ride home with Mike. He was driving an old loaner car because his Porsche was in the shop. As we pulled up to the top of our 100-yard uphill driveway, two men jumped out. They came to me at the passenger side and said, "Are you Mike?" When I replied in the affirmative, they pulled out a bunch of documents and slapped them on me. I feigned ignorance about their actions. Meanwhile, Mike Barch slipped out of the driver's side, went quietly in the house, down the stairs, and out the backdoor. He ran to the 10-foot fence and scurried over it and hid in the bamboo growing on the other side. I had figured out quickly who these guys were. They were most upset to find out I was Mike, but not Mike Barch.

One morning after I had left at 6:30, Mike left for the hospital and gave a ride to my future wife, a recovery room nurse. There was no talking to Rebecca until she had coffee. As she went to get in the car, Mike told her quietly to get in the car, buckle up, and hang on to her coffee. Mike had spotted a car blocking the bottom of our driveway with two men standing there. He then started down the driveway but took an immediate left across the large lawn of our next-door neighbor. Racing across the grass, mowing down saplings, tires spinning, he emerged from the partially wooded lawn down the road from the roadblock. Those smug guys started yelling and running after the car and disgustedly threw the legal papers at his car. My wife was holding on for dear life on this wild buggy ride. She liked to ease on into the day, not be taken for a rocket sled ride to work. The only thing missing was the *William Tell Overture* playing.

After Mike came home, I told him I would go with him to speak to our neighbor about making amends for the damage to the lawn and to corroborate his story. Our neighbor was a delightful guy, but to make matters worse, he was president of the Montgomery County Real Estate Association. He now had deep tire tracks all the way across his lawn and a slew of wasted saplings. We were very contrite, but he laughed very loudly when he heard the story and said not to worry about the damage. He would gladly take care of it and he was only sorry he did not witness foiling the process servers, no friends of his either. He loved us and would come by for a beer occasionally, but his wife did not particularly like us, there was way too much trouble to get into next door.

Winter in the Washington area was generally three months long and milder than the midwestern winters I had grown up with. Snow in Washington is catastrophic as people panic and scour the grocery stores to hoard toilet paper, bread, and other perishable items for fear of shortages. We never got much snow though one inch could paralyze the Washington area. Every five to ten years, however, we would get a substantial storm. One February while living in that house we got eighteen inches dumped on us. I was able to leave a bit early from the hospital and made it home fishtailing as I drove. No one was at our house and the 495 Beltway was shut down. A rare pristine silence blanketed the surrounding area. I hurriedly built a fire and began to prepare dinner. I had just sat down to enjoy a peaceful dinner when the loud noise of a large engine shattered the quiet. I went to our door and, lo and behold, there was Mike Barch driving a huge snowplow up our street. He had driven from downtown Washington to clear our neighborhood driveways with the huge industrial GW road grader snowplow! He warmed up by the fire, grabbed a plate of the chow, and then left to plow the street of his girlfriend, tooting the airhorn as he departed. It would have taken several days for the county to clear our street.

Meanwhile back downtown, the hospital was in a quandary. Employees understandably wanted to leave so they would not be stuck after a 12-hour overtime shift. The problem was that the next shift could not get in to work. Vital hospital functions required these employees to remain if possible. To entice them to stay, Mike instructed his staff to announce that an open bar with food would be available across the street for everyone who stayed. Many hospital employees stopped in after work.

The road to hell is paved with good intentions. Of course, the more it snowed, the more the liquor flowed. Several employees were overserved and now could not make it back across the street. Mike's assistants started a wheelchair taxi service and set up a "morgue" of several gurneys from the emergency room in the industrial work area of the hospital basement for them to sleep. They would be wheeled into the hospital elevators and checked in to their "hotel." I was told one guy was left by his escort with his head lolling and tongue out in the elevator thinking that someone would accept him in the basement. But that did not happen, and he kept riding up and down the elevator, opening up on patient floors. Somebody finally rescued him. Fortunately, both the employees and the hospital got back on their feet the next day.

Mike Barch's driving antics and general dynamic personality combined with a risk-taking mentality led his safety officer to start a betting pool on when Mr. Barch would kill himself with one of his stunts. He fooled them all and nobody collected.

But one day, that prophecy almost became reality, though not through any fault of his own. The safety officer burst in and exclaimed," Mike you must evacuate the hospital! There is a bomb in the east wing!" The safety officer, who had a chemistry background, said a maintenance man on the sixth floor was cleaning out an abandoned closet and where a large, capped glass bottle had crystals in the bottom where a liquid had evaporated. It obviously had been there awhile and forgotten. The label said it was a compound containing chlorine which he knew when dehydrated left a highly explosive residue that would go off if exposed to air or water or even jostled. He told everyone to freeze while he ran down to administration.

Mike elected to shut down the east wing and evacuate those patients. The Washington DC bomb squad was called and arrived in hazmat suits with a reinforced box for the bottle which was then put in the hazmat vehicle. They proceeded to take it to an FBI facility on an island in the Potomac River and the police detonated it creating a huge blast that left a large crater. The hospital literally dodged a huge bullet. Yikes, all that maintenance man had to do was bump that bottle with his broom.

Mike had GWU ready for major threats and problems. He had an arrangement with the Secret Service and FBI that if anything happened to the US president, he would be brought to GWU which was a Level One trauma center right downtown. Therefore, the destination was preordained the day President Reagan was shot at the Washington Hilton. Good friends working in the emergency room recall the red White House hotline ringing in the ER with the words, "The president is on his way to your place. He has been shot." He was brought to GWU and underwent emergency surgery in a well-documented saga, highlighted by the chief of surgery, my colleague and staunch Democrat Joe Giordano declaring, "Mr. President, today everyone is a Republican." Interestingly, my future wife was one of the ICU and recovery room nurses who helped care for President Reagan.

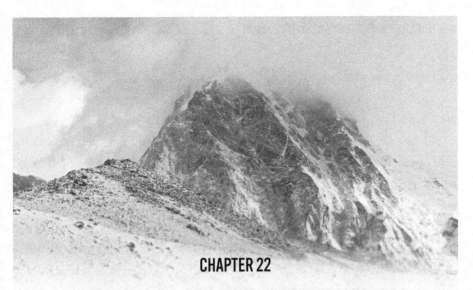

CHAPTER 22

NEW TECHNOLOGY OPENS DOORS

My clinical experience grew in conjunction with our practice which included two of my mentors, the chairman Harry Miller and our other partner, Said Karmi. All of us had different skills that complemented each other, and I thoroughly enjoyed working with them. Through the influence of Dr. Miller, I came to the attention of the American Urological Association (AUA) hierarchy for my training and work with lasers, a new tool in our armamentarium. While some could rightly say that a laser was a technology looking for an indication, I used various lasers for more than burning tissue. The establishment at GWU of the only NCI site outside of the NIH to treat bladder tumors with photodynamic therapy (PDT) demonstrated an entirely different use for lasers. In 1992, my interest in lasers and new technology led to me being asked to chair the AUA New Technology Committee which evaluated these medical advances and educated urologists globally on their proper use.

Technology in medicine exploded in the 1990s. Within ten years of my residency, the management of nearly 85 percent of urological problems changed, sometimes radically. Robotic surgery was introduced and underwent rapid transformation. New areas of minimally invasive surgical treatment were developed. New definitions were needed, hence the term "minimally invasive."

Other dramatic approaches were explored. Urinary stones could now be blasted from outside the body or retrieved through very small telescopes called endoscopes, laparoscopy developed from crude observation alone to a wide array of surgical applications and a new industry, an array of new or improved imaging technologies were introduced, dramatically increasing our ability to detect, treat, and monitor treatment effects for a variety of maladies. Cryotherapy (freezing tissue) began to be used for prostate cancer and other solid tumors. Virtual reality simulation was being used to train surgeons. Rapid advances in molecular biology were applied for diagnosis and development of new medications to attack diseases. Not only was I involved with their evaluation, but I was able to introduce them into our practice at GWU which then attracted patients from all over the U.S. and other countries for state-of-the-art medical care. In addition to the use of PDT and other laser technology at GWU, I was the first to perform laparoscopic surgery for urology in Washington DC with the removal of pelvic lymph nodes in prostate cancer. We shepherded the surgical robotic program at GW, also the first in Washington. We pioneered the use of imaging monoclonal antibodies for prostate cancer metastases. All these innovations put me in a prominent national position as a leader of new technology.

My interest in technology and background at NCI in optical physics led me to contact the Engineering Department at GWU to see how we could interact. They were delighted to have a clinician interested in applying engineering principles to medical problems. This type of collaboration is called translational research and I was appointed a Professor of Engineering in that department. We went on to explore early use of virtual reality to simulate surgery and train residents in the art of surgery. We published two papers on our techniques which were well received in the academic community as we demonstrated early on the value of virtual reality surgical simulation to teach the principles of endoscopy, the use of small telescopes, a hallmark of urological practice.

I branched out from there to evaluate other avant-garde imaging technologies such as optical coherent tomography (OCT) which used a different property of light to image tissue. Known as diffuse reflectance spectroscopy, this imaging used the differences between tissue layers and within tissue to create an image. If undetected abnormal tissue like in a tumor resided within normal tissue, you might be able to detect it with OCT by the way that it deflected light. This was particularly applicable for use with very aggressive small bladder tumors known as carcinoma in situ, mostly invisible to the naked eye, and we published our innovative data.

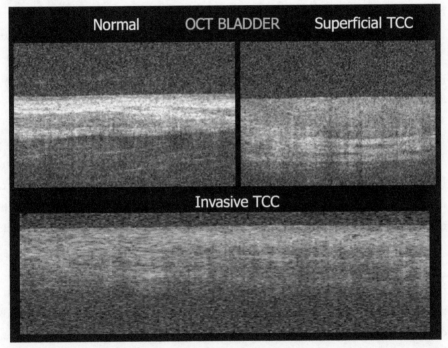

Optical Coherence Tomogaphy (OCT) imaging which delineates normal from abnormal bladder tissue. Clear tissue lines show no pathology, but cancer shows disruption of those interfaces.

As a corollary use of this technology, I had a discussion with anthropologist Dr. Bernard Wood, Professor of Human Origins at GWU. In his work on human evolution in conjunction with the Smithsonian, he was heavily involved with changes in teeth. We felt that OCT could be used to look at dental microanatomy and therefore differentiate between early human and early primate teeth. This noninvasive imaging was a novel way that successfully approached anatomical identification and it worked. This is what I mean about thinking outside of the box for research.

I was fortunate to be involved with the Director of the Human Origins program at the Smithsonian, Dr. Rick Potts, and his team of world class scientists. It is through him and his paleoanthropologist wife Jenny Clark, also a very close friend, that I am invited to the Smithsonian internal lectures. This also allowed me to revert to my original interests as a little kid!

GWU was very interested in all these technologies because the hospital could market its services in competitive markets. Consequently, Mike Barch, the VP of Medical Affairs, was very supportive of these new technologies in all disciplines.

Mike was interested in purchasing the type of laser I needed for PDT because he could parlay the collaboration with NCI into a significant marketing campaign. The laser company was in Germany and the manufacturer's representative wanted to send me to see someone treated in Italy and he agreed to have the administrator Mike Barch (who would purchase the equipment) accompany me. He was rather shocked to see how young my administrator was.

We met with the laser company owner in the picturesque medieval town Heroldsberg near Nuremberg, the second largest city in Bavaria. Since we went to Germany in August when all of Europe was on holiday, we found out that the case had been postponed. The laser company owner suggested we go to his chalet in Bavaria along with his daughter and her German princess friend.

While we were there, we went gliding in the Alps at a glider school. Essentially, these were very light aircraft without engines with nearly a mile long runway and a thick cord attached on one end to the nose and the other end to a V-8 GM auto engine. They revved the engine and the craft shot up in the air like a rollercoaster ride as one accelerated. Then the cord would drop off and you were 5000 feet in the air gliding down. The ride was quite a thrill at the beginning, like a rocket sled straight up, and then beautiful and smooth as the glider leveled out and you observed the postcard view except with the people moving. For all his bravado, my administrator was not as amused as I was. It was quite thrilling, and I returned several years later while speaking in Munich to try it again. We purchased the laser and started the NCI protocol at GWU.

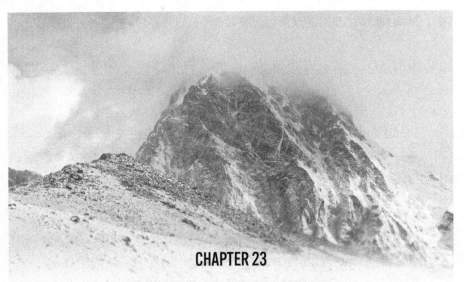

CHAPTER 23

BYZANTINE BAZAARS

Many other fascinating road trips materialized and because of my academic interests and research, I was invited to speak at several national and international conferences or as a visiting professor each year for many years. Often the hosts would arrange a visit of local interest for me and other times I would tack on a few extra days to catch a historical site or geographical highlight. For example, I was the featured speaker at a national medical conference at the 150-year-old British-established King Edward Medical University in Lahore, Pakistan, where I had lunch with the Governor of Punjab province. While I was there, the prominent urologist there asked me if I would consult on the case of a VIP government official. The Pakistani military chief of staff had prostate cancer and wanted a second opinion on his management. I reviewed everything with the 4-star general and made some recommendations for further care. He was most appreciative and offered to fly me in his private helicopter up to the spectacular Khyber Pass to view the cities of Quetta and Peshawar, areas that highly resisted the British during colonial days. I reluctantly had to decline because I was returning to the U. S. This is a trip I still regret missing.

> The old city in Lahore is a rabbit warren of small shops selling dry goods, spices, and exotic foods. One could easily disappear in this labyrinthine single lane bazaar that dates from the Middle Ages. Visitors are bombarded by merchants and varied pungent smells. I fully expected to run into Ali Baba. I purchased rugs in the bazaar sipping mint tea while viewing a dizzying array of carpets before haggling on the final price. It was not uncommon after extensive bargaining to think you got a pretty good deal only to find out that you may have a valuable rug, but your price still included a hefty profit for the rug merchant. These guys have been doing this for thousands of years, so you won't get anything over on them.

Speaking of bazaars, supposedly the original bazaar is the one in Istanbul which I visited with my wife when she accompanied me on a speaking engagement at an international congress in Rhodes, Greece. A side trip to Istanbul was memorable for carpet buying in the Grand Bazaar, for dinners on the Bosporus with medieval castles as background, visiting the Hagia Sofia and Topkapi Palace, and for a private boat tour of the Dardanelles Strait. Hiring that 30-seater boat by ourselves was punctuated by a humorous exchange with the Turkish boat captain who spoke no English. We were having a difficult time communicating when he brightened up and asked, "American?" When we acknowledged that we were indeed American, he beamed excitedly and proclaimed, "Ah, Monica Lewinsky!" How ironic and embarrassing that this man knew Monica Lewinsky but probably did not know we gave billions of dollars to the Turkish military each year.

On another occasion, I was the keynote speaker in Greece at the University of Athens for the annual "Athenian Days," a few days of academic presentations and discussion. My Greek guests put me up in the Athens Sheraton where I had perhaps the best view from any hotel I have ever stayed in because my window overlooked the Parthenon. A very unexpected turn of events ended the evening of the faculty dinner and after party at a large very modern music venue. As we were ready to leave, the urology chief resident tugged on my sleeve and told me that his professor, my host, had suggested that he take me somewhere special. It was now 1:30 in the morning and I had a morning flight back home, so I wondered what this was all about. We ended up at a very lively restaurant with a classical bouzouki band with people dancing on tables at 3 a.m. This slice of Greek life was thoroughly enjoyable, and I crawled out at 6 a.m. barely in time to dash to the hotel, jam my clothes in my suitcase, and get to the airport. I slept almost all the way home from Athens to Washington.

I have been fortunate to be an invited speaker twice at separate medical conferences in Egypt and Israel. In Cairo, my urologist host brought me to the Mena House where we lunched in the shadow of the Great Pyramid right next to the Sphinx. Besides this timeless view, the hotel was famous because it was the site of the 1977 Camp David Agreement, which restored Egypt's sovereignty over the Sinai peninsula. Another time in Jerusalem with my wife Rebecca, our guide was a professor of anthropology at Hebrew University and a most entertaining and knowledgeable escort. There was a miracle on every corner in Jerusalem and he punctuated his descriptions with pragmatic comments. For example, when we visited the supposed site of the Last Supper, he stated it could be the site but that the architecture style in that room was not introduced until the 4th century CE. He encouraged us to draw our own conclusions.

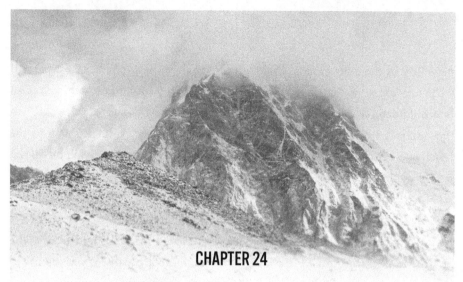

CHAPTER 24

THE MIDDLE EAST CONNECTION

I had exceptional training in kidney surgery with my mentor during residency and later partner, Dr. Said Karmi. He was both urology and transplant surgery board certified. Originally from Jordan, his father was an attorney/poet and the first ambassador to the United Nations from Jordan. Said had grown up as boyhood friends with King Hussein of Jordan. He became fast friends with Saudi Arabian ambassador Prince Bandar of Saudi Arabia. Said was a wonderful person and fantastic mentor for surgery and life, for that matter. He looked like Omar Sharif and had the old-world manners that endeared him to everyone. Said traveled often with Prince Bandar and his small entourage to London and the Middle East. This relationship led to a major collaboration between Saudi Arabia and GWU for medical education and hospital care that lasted years. For this collaboration, I was asked to review the urology services at King Faisal Specialist Hospital and spent a week in Riyadh.

I was often invited to join Said and his friends for lunch or dinner. His Middle East connections attracted notable international characters which included the American ambassador to Jordan, the principal lobbyist for the Palestine Liberation Organization (PLO headed by Yasser Arafat), Prince Bandar's director of security, the American legal counsel for the Saudis, the owner of the construction company that rebuilt Beirut's airport, prominent arms dealers, and occasionally members of the Saudi royal family and other diplomats. The discussions were fascinating and provided perspectives about the Middle East, not covered in mainstream media. Said and his association with the Saudis had provided a back channel for diplomatic discussions during the Gulf War for President George H. Bush.

The Saudi connection figured prominently in another interesting opportunity. GW got a new president, who was a pompous narcissistic attorney. He came in and immediately said that doctors had too much power in the university, and he was going to change that. My close friend Michael Barch who was the VP of Medical Affairs and ran the hospital saw the handwriting on the wall and departed for Johns Hopkins University as a dean. Over the course of several years, the president did not reinvest in the medical center, so it gradually became a very expensive enterprise. His solution was to put up the hospital for sale.

When the word got out about the sale, the usual corporate entities involved with hospital ownership like Universal Health were expected to be contenders to purchase GWU Medical Center. A small group of us, however, put together a consortium to bid. They included former GW Administrator Michael Barch, his top administrative assistant, my partner Dr. Said Karmi, and a couple of businessmen with corporate medical experience. The business plan we proposed was to create an international medical center that would cater to the diplomatic crowd. Nearly all countries have embassies in or near downtown Washington and proximity of their ambassadors and staff to first class medical care would be quite attractive. Our financial partners would be the Saudis and Said led the way to secure their financial backing for the $160 million bid which was $60 million greater than the next nearest bid. Our plans included marble floors and oriental rugs in the lobby and key public areas of the hospital, all single private rooms, accommodations and resources for security personnel, and other fixtures not often found in a hospital. GW already took care of many diplomats and had a small office that provided some support but there was no concerted effort to market and attract that population. We would truly make this an international medical center and magnet for that carriage trade.

The GW administration was blown away by the proposal, particularly so when they learned who was behind it, former and current GW people with the Saudis. Although there were political and social overtones to the Saudi involvement, the fact is that GW had quite a few Saudi students in undergraduate and graduate programs in addition to the contracted training of Saudi doctors in the medical center. Said and his association with the Saudis had provided a back channel for diplomatic discussions during the Gulf War for President George H. Bush. GW had an ongoing lucrative Saudi collaboration on health care. We were sure that the U.S. State Department would look favorably on such an institution since it would provide intelligence right in their backyard. GW is a few blocks from the State Dept headquarters.

Alas, it was not to be. The proposal was regarded as favorable by the Saudis and was on the desk of King Fahd to sign when he suffered an incapacitating stroke. With possible Saudi succession to the throne looming and with the jockeying of the royal hierarchy for favorable position, it was felt to be too delicate politically to proceed. The proposal was tabled on the Saudi side pending possible rearrangement of their government. This now indefinite delay forced GW to consider the other purchase proposals and they accepted the second-best bid for $100 million to build a new hospital in a corporate partnership. Our group has often thought about the irony surrounding these events. But for an ill-timed blood clot, we would have created an international medical center which would present many opportunities for growth and income. I would likely have been the medical director, at least for the transition, and the trajectory of my professional (and likely private) life would have been redirected.

This connection with the Saudis led to a very interesting consultation. Jim Marinucci is an emergency medical technician and experienced wound care specialist who was the liaison for GW international medical programs. Jim asked me in 2009 if I could consult for a Saudi royal family member. Jim was not sure what the problem was, but the royal family had requested a urologist and would not elaborate. After I agreed I found out that I was to head a medical contingent to deal with someone very high in the royal family. Since health care issues are held close to the vest for high government officials in nearly all countries, we could only speculate.

I flew to a private clinic in Geneva with other seasoned MDs from GW. Upon landing, I was taken right away to the royal family head physician. I had been expecting the medical issue to be something relatively common like urinary difficulties from prostate enlargement, prostate cancer, or erectile dysfunction. I was quite surprised to learn that the patient was the Saudi Crown Prince Sultan, brother to King Abdullah and heir to the throne. Furthermore, after reviewing his CT scan provided to me upon arrival in Saudi Arabia, it became apparent that the problem was quite complex. He had congenital anomaly known as a horseshoe kidney, a rare condition that occurs when the two kidneys do not separate in the pelvis as usual in utero. Horseshoe kidneys come with multiple attendant anatomic aberrations. His royal majesty had bilateral obstruction of his kidneys. This is the type of case that you would discuss with a panel of urologists but was now just dumped in my lap.

We met with more than twenty consulting physicians and multiple royal family members. Test results were shared and then an opinion was offered by each physician in turn. I was last and listened intently as everyone gave their opinion. When it was my turn to speak, I thanked all for their comments but that the real problem was retroperitoneal fibrosis, scar tissue that pulled both ureters medially causing bilateral urinary obstruction in the pelvis. Both ureters were partially obstructed but to leave that situation would invite deterioration of the solitary kidney unit. Everybody looked astounded, they had missed the diagnosis, but I had pegged it. I explained that retroperitoneal fibrosis is scar tissue that can be caused by a few different things. One is abdominal cancer; another is a leaking aortic aneurysm. Some medications are very rarely known to do this and use of LSD can cause this. I was NOT going to suggest that the Crown Prince had been using LSD. The Crown Prince was beloved by his people. The next day we finally learned that the prince had a colon resection for cancer four years ago. This meant it was likely the cancer in the pelvis had recurred.

Before the prince went into colonoscopy for evaluation the next day, I spoke to him directly. I told him not to worry, he would sail through this, and we would get some answers. Holding my hand with both of his, he smiled gratefully at me, looking into my eyes, and said emphatically, 'I know you will take care of me."

The biopsy of a suspicious area suggested the cause of obstruction. Our entourage departed on a customized 747 with all business class seats for Agadir, Morocco, a resort city on the Atlantic Ocean where the Saudis maintained a magnificent palace. The medical team was quartered in an upscale hotel near the palace where the Crown Prince was recovering. The Saudis used this palace as a surrogate capital during summer every year. They had 300 Mercedes cars, and each of us was given a car and driver. The palace was truly elegant with museum quality Islamic engraving in gold and silver all over the huge walls and stunning Persian rugs on top of the marble floors, all with a panoramic view of the Atlantic. At the palace we would all assemble to drink tea and hear the daily lab results and get an update on the prince's condition to make recommendations. After our daily meeting, we were free to go back to the hotel.

One night shortly after the procedure for the prince, we were at dinner, enjoying cigars at a beachfront restaurant when we got an urgent call from the palace. The prince was having a fever spike and was restless, a possible sign of impending systemic infection. We mobilized the whole team and raced at nearly 100 mph through the small town to the palace. I thought we were going to die in a motor vehicle accident on the way there, which took all of five minutes.

There were thirty or forty lesser princes standing around in robes and kaffiyehs. A few of us were brought into the prince's bedroom where he was in his pajamas. I wondered to myself just how many westerners had met the prince in his jammies. He needed an intravenous catheter, and our expert ICU physician got a small but sufficient vein on the first shot.

The prince recovered and we departed four days later. I told the lead physician that they had to relieve the bilateral ureteral obstruction which would require an abdominal procedure. I explained that I could do this rare procedure but that I would ask a close friend and world-renowned reconstructive urologist to join me. Because of the implications of recurrent colon cancer, he also needed to be in a major medical center. Considering all of this, I had suggested one of three places, MD Anderson Cancer Center in Houston, Memorial Sloan Kettering Cancer Center, or Cornell in New York, or we could do this in Washington.

I returned to Washington and contacted a close friend, Dave McLeod, chair of urology at Walter Reed Army Medical Center. I explained the problem and asked if we could use the suite reserved for the U.S. president at Walter Reed. He suggested we tour the suite. It was ideal with a secluded private entrance and elevator and a large suite with marble floors, Persian rugs, and museum quality paintings. It also had significant facilities for security. We received permission to use the suite for this head of state. The royal family huddled up and then decided to go to Cornell where close friends of mine performed the operation and kept me appraised. I was told that the Saudis preferred not to be in Washington to downplay the significance which had international policy implications. The successful surgery at Cornell for the Crown Prince confirmed the recurrence of colon cancer. Unfortunately, the prince died several years later from this problem.

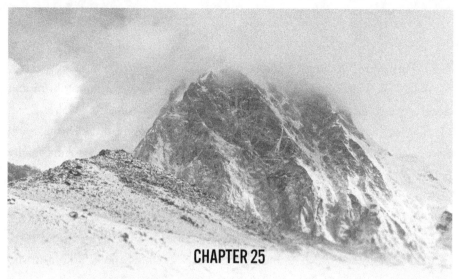

CHAPTER 25

AN UNUSUAL CLINICAL PRACTICE

There are many stories about some of the famous and infamous patients who came for urological issues including presidential candidates, White House cabinet members and staff, the vice president, the controversial mayor of Washington, early civil rights leaders, diplomats and ambassadors from many countries, celebrities, and other people in the news. For example, Bob Barker used to fly in from Los Angeles to see me.

One day, the controversial mayor of Washington Marion Barry was referred to me for an elevation of a blood test known as prostate specific antigen (PSA) which could signify prostate cancer. Mr. Barry was a very prominent early civil rights leader who parlayed that into becoming the Washington, DC, mayor for several terms. While there were very justified rumors of corruption in his administration, he avoided any problems until he was caught smoking crack cocaine and went to jail. Now he was out of jail and re-elected as mayor. The repeated level of PSA elevation dictated that a prostate biopsy be performed but he would not respond for a repeat visit to discuss and explain this. Therefore, a registered letter was sent to which he reluctantly replied and returned. If we did not follow this path, the patient could claim he never received the information. You can imagine the uproar that would cause with racial overtones.

Mr. Barry was an interesting character. Educated as a chemist, he entered politics early and never looked back. His wife at the time I met him was the Washington boxing commissioner, an occupation with suspect legal activity associated with it. At first angry and suspicious, he gradually came to appreciate me over the course of our interaction which was shaky due to non-compliance with medical care at times. We ended up with an amicable relationship, but it took a while.

Marion's biopsy unfortunately came back positive for prostate cancer. Now we had to talk about the approach for treatment. I had just reviewed the data for the accuracy of a brand-new scan to evaluate the most likely source of possible spread, the pelvic lymph nodes, one that employed a small radioactive particle attached to a very specific antibody for prostate cancer. The negative predictive value was 92 percent, meaning if the scan was negative, 92 percent of the time that was accurate and no cancer was in the lymph nodes. I was an investigator for this study and an author on the pending publication. These were quite good results and had not been published yet. I recommended the scan with the thought that if it was positive in the area of lymph nodes, we could sample them by laparoscopy. If negative, I felt comfortable recommending definitive treatment by surgical removal of the prostate or radiation. If positive lymph nodes or distant areas of activity were found, a different systemic approach would be necessary. His scan was negative, so he had a chance for treatment of the prostate for cure.

Compounding his health management was how to manage the publicity and public relations around this discovery. The announcement was national news as you can imagine. Marion asked me to be at the press conference with him on stage when the diagnosis was announced and the national press was there in force. I had to laugh when friends told me later they couldn't figure out at first who the big white bodyguard was with Marion Barry but it was his doctor, me. Once we answered questions for the audience, I was besieged off stage by live news reporters. I told them I would answer their questions but not any questions about the mayor's personal data. Of course, at least one reporter ambushed me to ask what the PSA level was and other personal information. My reply was that you had better ask Mr. Barry himself because I could not divulge that information. We had to pay attention when the media are involved.

Mr. Barry went on to have successful surgery to remove his prostate and his lymph nodes were negative for malignancy. Over his postoperative course we had to deal with a few issues and some non-compliant patient behavior, but he fared rather well overall. He actually was surprisingly very supportive of our research efforts and showed up unannounced with full press entourage to a reception Steve Patierno and I held in the GWU Hospital lobby to promote prostate cancer research. He also asked me to join him for a series of televised press conferences throughout the city to promote men getting their PSA levels checked. He really was a chameleon.

One of the interesting outcomes of this saga with Marion Barry was that some African American patients started coming in who had been involved in the early civil rights movement. They would typically say that they had seen I had taken care of Marion Barry and that drew them in. Courtland Cox was the quiet legal brain behind the Student Non-violent Coordinating Center (SNCC) which was a hotbed of racial activity and dedicated to empower disenfranchised African Americans in the Jim Crow south. He actually was one of the few patients who became a personal friend and I used to run into him in town. He is a true gentleman whom I had to treat with a complicated surgical situation. Stokely Carmichael who led SNCC back in the day contacted me to consult with him on his prostate cancer which was unfortunately already advanced. In fact, there was a great book *Dream City* about the Washington civil rights history authored by Tom Sherwood and Harry Jaffe which detailed the roles of several other patients of mine in its history. Tom was the primary News 4 TV reporter and Harry was the senior editor of Washingtonian Magazine. I was interviewed by Tom on multiple occasions over the years with significant activity around the time of Marion Barry's management. Harry also interviewed me for some Washingtonian pieces including one I am very proud of, *The 50 Best and Brightest of Washington* where I was chosen for inclusion because of my academic career and extracurricular activities related to expedition medicine. That was quite an honor.

Another time we held a conference about prostate cancer detection and treatment and were honored to have Senator Bob Dole, former Senate majority leader and at the time presidential candidate, to speak about the need for detection. His surgeon and good friend of mine, Colonel Dave McLeod at Walter Reed, was internationally known for his prostate cancer research and treatment.

I helped Dave once a week in his clinic. Dave had operated on some famous people related to the military including several senators, commander of the Desert Storm Gulf War General Schwarzkopf, and others. Dave was a big practical joker and I had been the brunt of his humor a few times. One day in the clinic, I overheard an upset Dave McLeod really giving it to his staff for not notifying him of a VIP patient, saying he really needs to see those people and that he would fire people who did not notify him. Ha, I saw an opportunity for payback. A week or so later, Dave was out on the ward in the hospital. I went into his office and taped a short note to his computer that said, "Hi Dave, came by to see you, where the h**l were you? Bob Dole." When I came back the next week, I innocently said I heard Senator Dole was in last week. Of course, the staff had not seen Senator Dole, he was never there. They told me Dr. McLeod really got upset , yelled at everybody, and threatened to fire the whole lot on the spot. I finally told Dave that I was the culprit so he wouldn't be angry at his staff, knowing I was back in his crosshairs.

Several years later, I took my daughter Rachel to our favorite watering hole in downtown Washington, the Prime Rib. This classic steakhouse was a powerhouse gathering place for diplomats and celebrities. My son Tim worked there as a busboy when he first got out of high school and said the US Secret Service would come there regularly to make a sweep and check that emergency entrances were clear because of the clientele. When Rachel and I sat at the bar, a gentleman on my other side struck up a conversation where I learned that he was a private nurse taking care of a VIP who was at a table. He told me it was Senator Bob Dole and I responded that I knew the Senator though had not seen him in several years but please give him my regards, he might remember me. A short time later, the nurse came back and said Senator Dole certainly did remember me and invited us to his table. Rachel and I joined his table which had his chief of staff and that of Vice President Pence. After we sat down, I told him I had a story to tell him about Dave McLeod and related what happened when I left a note supposedly from him to Dave. Senator Dole laughed very loudly and thoroughly enjoyed the story, Dave McLeod's reputation was well known.

Proximity to the White House brought others in for medical consultation, some of them seen on the national nightly news. One day I received a call from a close friend and partner in a large multinational law firm, Skadden, Arps, Slate, Meagher, & Flom LLP. He was working closely with a senior partner, Bob Bennett, who was representing President Bill Clinton in the sexual harassment lawsuits brought by Jennifer Flowers and Paula Jones. One of the important components in the Paula Jones case was the fact that she claimed she could identify a very private physical trait of the president. Without getting into explicit details, the attorneys wanted what is known as an independent medical evaluation (IME) for confirmation of this condition. My friend wanted to know if I could discretely examine the president and prepare a report for them. What a grenade was lobbed into my lap! My role may be central to this entire case and whatever was found, I would be in the crosshairs of one side or the other. Not that I had anything to hide, but serious scrutiny would be paid to my background and perhaps skewed to tarnish my reputation. I told him that I probably could do an IME but would need to think about it. I figured I may need legal counsel to protect myself, regardless of my friend. While I mulled this quandary, the scene shifted dramatically with the Monica Lewinsky story that bubbled up, relegating the Paula Jones case at least temporarily to the back burner. I think I dodged a bullet though I do not know which side would have fired.

An interesting patient, Ambassador Joseph Wilson, came to see me in consultation. It turned out, the ambassador had been assigned to several countries in Africa and we had mutual associates. After his evaluation, we kept in touch for a while, exploring whether there was common ground to work together on African healthcare issues. His wife, Valerie Plame, came in with him. At that time, she was a CIA officer. She was the subject of the 2003 Plame affair, also known as the CIA leak scandal. Plame's identity as a CIA officer was disclosed and subsequently published by of *The Washington Post*.

In the aftermath of the scandal, Richard Armitage was identified as one source of the information. Armitage was a senior mentor of my close friend Scott Harrison. Scooter Libby, Chief of Staff to Vice President Dick Cheney, was convicted of lying to investigators. After a failed appeal, President Bush commuted Libby's sentence and in 2018, President Trump pardoned him. No one was formally charged with leaking the information.

Plame wrote a with a ghostwriter detailing her career and the events leading up to her resignation from the CIA. She has published at least two spy novels. A 2010 biographical feature film, *Fair Game*, was produced based on memoirs by her and her husband.

I always asked where a patient was from and what they did. One day, a patient in my clinic told me he was from Christchurch, New Zealand. When I asked why he was here from such a distant land, he told me, "Because my daughter married a pervert." When following up on this peculiar answer with further information, it dawned on me. There had been a sensational story of a plastic surgeon who claimed her daughter was being sexually abused by her physician husband and then the daughter disappeared. It turned out that she had been sent accompanied by her grandfather on a circuitous route to a country without an extradition treaty with the US and speculation was that the former intelligence agent grandfather was responsible. William Morgan, an older rather rotund gent with full white beard who would be a perfect model for Santa Claus, was the grandfather now in my office. He told me the details of the case and how the court dismissed the facts, but he was adamant, with good justification. He assured me the granddaughter was now safe. He had a fascinating background as an OSS agent (forerunner of the CIA) in World War II who had parachuted into Nazi-occupied France and fought with the resistance. He then joined the Eisenhower administration in the White House as a psychological operations expert and was involved with thwarting Russian objectives against the West. He gave me a very interesting book about his life which still adorns my bookshelf.

One of the good guys was the deputy chief of mission for the Indonesian embassy, who came in for regular checkups every six months. One day he told me he regretted that this was the last time he would see me because he was being transferred. He had just been named Indonesian ambassador to the Vatican. I told him that was wonderful, congratulations, and that maybe I would see him one day in Rome. A year later I was an invited speaker for an international medical conference in Milan and I contacted the ambassador and he said he would be delighted to have me as his guest in Rome and I was invited to stay at the ambassadorial mansion with his family. He picked me up in a huge, escorted limo with Indonesian flags flying above the headlights and transported me to the massive ambassadorial residence.

My Notre Dame close friend Phil Brady in the Bush White House urged me to contact his friend and U.S. ambassador to the Vatican, Tom Milady. The friendly ambassador invited me to the annual Fourth of July party held at his residence that week. When I got back to the Indonesian residence, my ambassador friend pulled me aside and gave me a present, the large medal he received from the Pope upon presenting his credentials to the Vatican. He said he knew I was Catholic so it might be more significant to me than it was to him, a Muslim. I was very touched and said I did not want to take his keepsake, but he insisted. Then he said he wanted me to go with him to the US embassy for the Fourth of July celebration. He was quite surprised when I told him Ambassador Milady had already invited me and I would be delighted to accompany him.

The U.S. ambassador's residence was an ancient Roman villa with a large garden in the back filled with priceless archaeological Roman statues and busts on pedestals. There were roughly one hundred guests with twenty cardinals in their red robes and skull caps. There were several ambassadors from other countries there. That's why many guests were addressed as "Excellency" as that was the mode of address for both ambassadors and cardinals. A group of them had a good laugh when I pronounced that my only title was doctor and certainly not "Excellency" like all the rest of them.

I was now a Professor of Urology and Engineering and was offered a professorship in the Department of Immunology, Microbiology, and Tropical Medicine by chairman Dr. Peter Hotez, later a 2022 Nobel Prize candidate for his development of a novel and affordable COVID-19 vaccine. I make no claims to be an expert in immunology, but I certainly have experience in all the others. It is a strange assortment of titles and positions. I have not run into anyone else with that combination. My interests in urology, technology, and tropical medicine do share a common thread.

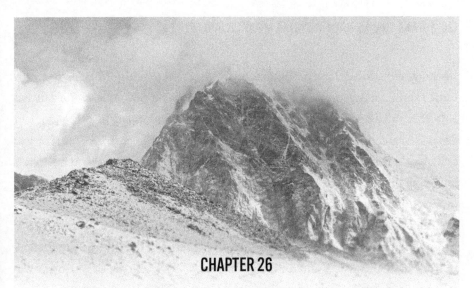

CHAPTER 26

AEROSPACE MEDICINE WITH NASA

R elatively early in my career, I was asked along with several other physicians from different disciplines and hospitals in the region to attend a meeting sponsored by NASA to discuss medical applications for diagnosis and treatment while in space. The leaders of the meeting were scientists and administrators from the large NASA Ames Research Center in northern California. They addressed the meeting by saying they wanted to design something like the Star Trek tri-corder which could diagnose disease by sweeping it over the person to be evaluated. They asked what information should be collected and the usual and rather obvious answers came up: blood pressure, temperature, oxygen saturation, and body chemistry.

I finally raised my hand and said that diagnostic light technology would be very useful. I then explained that light had four properties in tissue: it can be transmitted, reflected, absorbed, or scattered. Depending on the light source and intensity, each one of these noninvasive approaches would provide information about the scanned tissue. I explained that in my laser work at the National Cancer

Institute, we used all those properties. As I walked out to return to work, two men came running down the aisle to intercept me. They said they were senior officials at NASA and asked me to present my thoughts and participate in a think tank at Ames Research Center in California. That meeting was fascinating in that I was one of only three physicians among about fifty other major scientist participants including physicists, materials scientists, chemists, molecular biologists, radiation experts, meteorologists, and other specialists.

That meeting launched several years of intriguing collaboration with NASA. Around that time, I was contacted by Dr. Rich Williams, the chief medical officer (CMO) of NASA who wanted to send some NASA VIPs to me as patients. I was asked to join the Aerospace Medicine and Occupational Health Advisory Committee (AMOHAC) which oversaw the health and welfare of U. S. astronauts and their families. At the first committee meeting, which was attended by many people not on the committee, it was obvious that, although I had strong credentials, the other members had a greater breadth of experience. There were military surgeon generals, heads of national medicine institutes, and the like. I asked Dr. Williams why he wanted me on this committee, and he told me I was the only committee member who had medical evacuation experience in the civilian sector and my perspective was desired.

Over the course of the next four years, we created policies for our astronauts and published scientific papers on risk related to space travel. There are problems unique to space travel that concern NASA such as more intense radiation and a corresponding need for astronaut protection. Microgravity causes expansion of the cardiac chambers. Effects on equilibrium can be chronic from high G forces in flight. Dr. Williams was an experimental aircraft pilot and a USAF flight surgeon with experience in fighter aircraft in addition to being a surgeon and discovered and published a syndrome related to gravitational effects on the inner ear where equilibrium regulation occurs.

My time spent with NASA was fascinating and Dr. Williams remains a very good friend. I am proud to have sponsored him as a fellow in The Explorers Club.

A few years later, I was invited to attend the NASA New Horizons program Pluto Flyby by Dr. Alan Stern, the project principal investigator. This voyage to the only unexplored planet in the Solar System intended to understand the formation of the Plutonian system, the Kuiper belt, and the transformation of the early Solar System. The spacecraft collected data on the atmospheres, surfaces, interiors, and environments of Pluto and its moons. Our spacecraft passed by Pluto after a near decade long journey on July 14, 2015, to much fanfare and international press. Alan told me there were several Eagles among the senior staff of the program including himself. The photos with all of us cheering were shared with the national Boy Scout and Eagle Scout organizations for their websites and publications that went out to the millions of scouts.

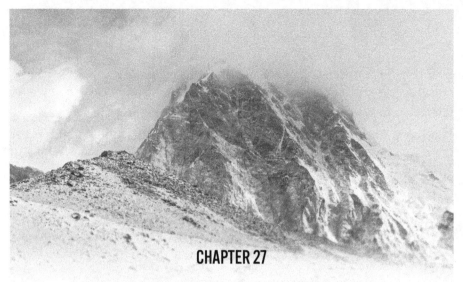

FASCINATING LAB DISCOVERY AND VENOMOUS SNAKES

At GWU, I was fortunate to sit on a research committee with a young basic science PhD researcher with similar interests. This began over a decade of research that led to ten patents and several professional publications.

Dr. Steve Patierno and I met to discuss what I had been working on at NCI. He was immediately attracted to my work with a protein called uteroglobin (UG) because it was first described in the uterus of a pregnant rabbit. Although consequently identified in other animal tissues, I was looking for a similar system in the human prostate along with a key scientist in that area. Uteroglobin inhibited the very basic mechanism of inflammation, a cascade of biochemical events, involving phospholipase A2 (PLA2). Activation of PLA2 is the first step in inflammation. If you block PLA2, it stops this cascade of biochemical reactions that end in inflammation. One could therefore shut down inflammation. This had implications for many disease states in which experts believed inflammation was a component such as arthritis, cystic fibrosis, chronic infections, and asthma, to name a few. Steve told me this was very interesting to him because of a possible role in cancer metabolism.

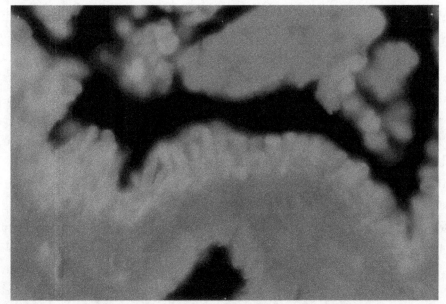

Uteroglobin (UG) is a protein produced in the epithelial lining of many organs. UG blocks the first step of inflammation that, when lost as cancer develops, promotes metastasis to occur.

Steve called me a couple of weeks later and said that UG shuts down the first step of metastasis which is invasion of the cancer cell into the surrounding tissue as a precursor to distant spread. When I saw the experimental data later, it was indeed breathtaking. We quickly met to plot the next steps.

If this was to be further developed, it would require significant investment of time and resources. Funding could come from agencies like the NCI but that would likely be limited and highly competitive since there are many groups seeking such support. If private sources of funding were sought, we had to control the narrative and direction of research. In either case, control would accrue to who had the rights. Therefore, we formed a small company dedicated to further development of UG for cancer. We had to file patents, but UG was already in the public domain because of earlier research on inflammation so the only patents we could apply for are known as use patents, basically the use of the invention for stated purposes. The first step was to get the right to patent our findings from the university since we were both employees and GWU essentially owned our rights. Metastatin Pharmaceuticals was born with seed money from all the principals. After about a year while we collectively held our breath, our attorney finally negotiated a very favorable agreement for the rights from GW which retained a small portion of equity.

To develop the Metastatin product would require about $5 million dollars to get through preclinical work and preliminary human testing. We received more than $1 million in chunks over the next two years, which allowed us to continue research. Because UG was made in nearly all tissues with an epithelial lining (mouth, throat, lungs, intestine, prostate, endometrium, bladder) replacement UG would not be toxic at all. Essentially, UG is made in normal tissue but as that tissue became cancerous, UG expression was lost. This allowed the now cancerous cells to escape the local environment and metastasize. Therefore, the braking system for cancer spread was removed. It is metastasis that kills people, usually not the primary tumor. Replacing UG in those cancerous tissues became our goal.

Our research further showed the same process in other tumors originating in lung, uterine, head and neck, esophagus, and colon and we consequently applied for patents to cover use of UG in those types of tumors. But after five years trying to raise money and failing to attract a large partner with proper resources, we had to disband the company and shut down our efforts. This is the fate of many small biotech companies due to lack of funding. We still cannot find a flaw in our logic or science and firmly believe that this system will be investigated again for its role in cancer metabolism. I still dream about the potential contribution to medicine that was not realized.

Years later this topic surfaced again. Watching a zoom presentation from The Explorers Club, one of the speakers was working in the field of envenomation. The company the speaker founded, Ophirex, is a developer of a toxin-targeting antidote called varespladib designed for snakebite to help the 500,000 people who die or suffer amputations each year from venomous snakebite. About 70 percent of those who die never even make it to the hospital for treatment. The antidote is a small molecule therapy for snakebite victims intended for worldwide human and veterinary use, with an oral formulation for use in the field, where most bites occur, enabling doctors to get safe, effective, and accessible initial treatment for snakebite envenoming. Current antidotes, if even available, are quite expensive and require stringent conditions to store. The Ophirex product comes in tablet as well as intravenous formulation.

In the middle of the presentation, Dr. Matt Lewin, the speaker stated that the system he was working with involved blocking activation of PLA2. I sat up immediately and paid attention. What they had developed is a tablet or intravenous compound that shuts down inflammation which was responsible for the effects in envenomation. This is a major accomplishment that would allow widespread as well as remote use.

In the U.S., 11,000 people are bitten annually by venomous snakes with about five deaths but the annual global toll for snakebites is greater than 125,000 deaths and 400,000 permanent disabilities.

I contacted Dr. Lewin a couple of days later and stated my background in PLA2 research. He was astounded, telling me he had only run into one other person who knew about this system in some detail. Ophirex had overcome a major obstacle that we had encountered, namely, how to make this product practical to be used as a medicine. I was very excited and told him he should also look at its use for cancer and arthritides in addition to envenomation which was huge on its own. Ophirex had done a great job in obtaining funding and proprietary rights through a patent portfolio and they took the correct approach to develop one indication and make that a viable product with proper study. You need to pull this across the goal line before you go on to develop other indications.

The varespladib product is now in clinical trials for venomous snakebites and he sent me a video of a pig that had been injected with krait venom, a deadly snake in South Asia. The pig had been injected with three times the amount of venom needed to kill an adult human. As the pig was lying there with agonal breathing, essentially dying, it was injected with varespladib, and twenty minutes later it was running around the cage like nothing happened. It was amazing! I am very excited to see further development of this product and its use in other conditions.

Constrictors and venomous snakes have reared their heads throughout my career in various circumstances. When I was a resident on call, I received a page from the emergency room. It was the ER doc who told me that there was a patient who needed to be admitted to the hospital and he thought he should go on our service because he had blood in his urine. That could be an indication for admission to the urology service, but I needed more information to make that decision. I asked the circumstances leading to his seeking the ER. Was there flank pain or pain on urination? Difficulty with urination? Did he have a fever? Any medical history that might contribute such as a coagulation defect or sickle cell disease? The ER doc then said he had sustained a snakebite the previous day and his index finger was very swollen. I asked if they identified the type of snake, but they had not. Then I told the ER doc that he was probably bitten by a copperhead or possibly a rattlesnake and that he had hemolysis (red blood cells breaking up) from the snake hemotoxin with leakage into his urine of the hemoglobin components. I said thanks, interesting case, but no admission to urology, we will be glad to see him as a consultant. We will watch over your shoulder. The doctor had called someone who knew something about venomous snakebites.

When I was a resident on rotation at Children's National Medical Center, we were consulted when a teenager broke into the herpetarium at the National Zoo and decided to steal a pretty, thick, multicolored snake. He had brought a burlap sack to toss whatever he stole and got the snake into the bag and threw it over his shoulder. Of course, the snake struck, and this teenager flagged down a city bus and said he needed to go to the hospital because he thought he had been bitten by a venomous snake. When evaluated there, the personnel there discovered the bite and immediately called the zoo. They learned that a very venomous snake had been stolen, the Gaboon Viper. Fortunately, the zoo had the antivenin for this viper, and it was rushed over to Childrens Hospital National Medical Center. The patient nearly died and lost his kidney function. The snake survived but was so traumatized that it was sequestered for over a year.

There were some nasty snakes in the areas where I traveled. There are several dangerous ones in Africa. My good South African friend and colleague at GlaxoSmithKline, James van Hasselt, is also a urologist with similar interests to mine. He told me a story from his friend, the doctor at the clinic in Kruger National Park. The clinic doctor was called by a rancher in the bush who had just been bitten by an unidentified snake but feared it was a deadly black mamba. The doc loaded up a large amount of mamba antivenin and left on an emergency flight immediately. Upon arriving, the rancher walked out to the plane and said he was doing fine. The doc, however, noted some slurring of words and he immediately put the man on a stretcher, started an IV, and gave him a large dose of antivenin. The rancher had begun to complain of losing feeling in his legs and that it was ascending. Shortly after the antidote was given, he felt better and said the feeling had returned to his legs. But, halfway to the hospital in the plane, he started to complain of ascending numbness. This snake has a neurotoxin which, if it reaches the diaphragm, will paralyze his breathing, causing death.

The doctor called ahead for an ambulance and told the medics to be ready to intubate the patient. Immediately upon landing, they rushed him onto a stretcher and immediately put the tube in his throat so they could control his breathing. He also administered the rest of the antivenin. This patient did survive in the nick of time, but many others are not so lucky in the bush.

Speaking of mambas, James sent me a video from his cousin who lived on a farm in South Africa on a nature conservancy. The video showed a huge black mamba crawling out of the trellis above the doorway to his cottage. The riveting video showed foot after foot of the snake emerging and crawling down the front of the house to the ground…and then curling around the bare foot of his cousin before slowly going off into the grass. This mamba was 13 feet long, the largest they had ever seen. Fortunately, it was habituated to his cousin so did not bother him. I held my breath just watching this incredible video. Whew!

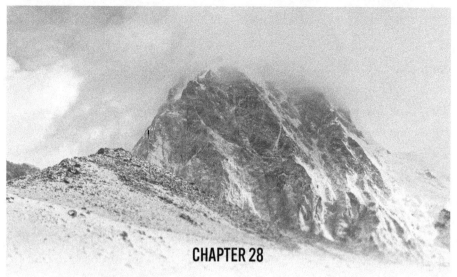

CHAPTER 28

DRAGGING ME BACK IN THE TENT

I was speaking at the Boy Scouts of America (BSA) national jamboree at Fort A. P. Hill when President George W. Bush was scheduled to speak as well. It was a really sweltering day in Virginia of 103°. Severe thunderstorms and tornado warnings cancelled the president just before he was to speak. He was rescheduled to return for the closing ceremony, and he was scheduled to speak right before my appearance. The theme for the week-long events for the Boy Scouts was exploration and I had received a strange letter from BSA saying I had been selected to have a camp named for me because I was a living explorer and Eagle Scout. Thinking this was a humorous joke (I do have prankster friends who probably owed me one or two), I called BSA headquarters and found out they were quite serious. I was quite blown away. My camp was to hold 1600 Boy Scouts from the New York area and came complete with a huge flag with a personal logo and emblazoned with "Camp Michael Manyak." This was a great honor! I had been out of scouting for forty years. There were other camps named for notable Eagle Scouts, like astronauts, titans of business, and explorers who had been the deepest in the ocean and who had parachuted from the stratosphere. BSA had created a deck of cards with a card for each of us with a photo and our exploits listed. Scouts were encouraged to identify us and get as many autographs as they could.

When I arrived, I had a senior scout executive handler who shuttled me around to various events, interviews, and to other camps to meet leaders and scouts. I had to sign autographs all over the place and people brought their sons up to meet me. I met a lot of fine young men who were quite accomplished already. The weeklong series of events and activities was very humbling.

Because the theme was Living Explorers, the BSA wanted us to lead the final ceremony which now had speakers from the cancelled opening ceremony. With a backdrop of The Explorers Club headquarters projected (a spectacular place like a museum) complete with elephant tusks and Admiral Perry's sled, the president of the Club Richard Wiese and I ran the show, sending some selected Boy Scouts on an imagined expedition. President Bush gave a great presentation right before our show. From the stage, the attendees seemed endless and later, I learned that some 90,000 people were there.

During the week at the jamboree, I ran into a good friend from The Explorers Club whom I had known for about ten years. Bill Steele is a world class speleologist (cave scientist) and has won every award available in that scientific community. When I asked what he was doing at the jamboree, he told me he was president of the National Eagle Scout Association (NESA). Soon after, Bill asked me to join the board of directors. This led to a very productive and current collaboration when I created the NESA World Explorers program. This program is now distinctive for sending nationally-selected Eagle Scouts on expeditions to the Amazon, Galapagos, dinosaur digs, Yellowstone to work with NASA, a survival camp in Puerto Rico run by Special Forces members, an ongoing bald eagle survey in northern Michigan to evaluate effects of pollution, paleoanthropology in South Africa with a newly-discovered human species, speleology in Mammoth Cave, and to the Arctic to work with narwhals.

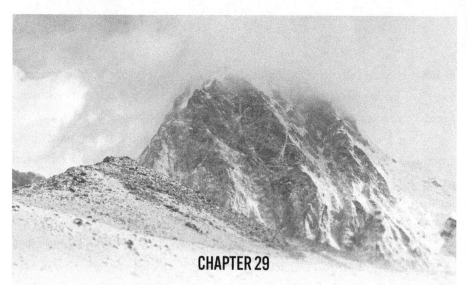

CHAPTER 29

CRYPTOZOOLOGY AND THE EXPLORERS CLUB

While conducting clinical and research work as well as consulting, I still made time for my passion for exploration.

I ran across an article about a small group of explorers called The International Society of Cryptozoology. I called the secretary of the society, Richard Greenwell, and we spoke at length about his expedition to the Congo River Basin looking for a large unknown animal rumored to exist there. He agreed that a doctor with tropical medicine experience would be quite useful in such a remote, hostile environment. He put me in touch with the society president, Dr. Roy Mackal, who also had claimed to have seen the Loch Ness monster, a dubious claim without substantiation. Then Richard Greenwell asked if I was near the University of Maryland. They were having their board of directors meeting there very soon and I was invited as a guest. That colorful meeting had noted biological scientists in their midst as well as the sasquatch and Loch Ness monster hunters. The next time I saw noted anthropologist and foremost sasquatch expert Grover Krantz was in the Smithsonian where his skeleton and that of his pet Irish wolfhound were mounted in an exhibit on osteology. He had willed his body to the Smithsonian. Strange indeed.

After this meeting, I was asked to become the group's Field Medical Advisor for their member constituents as a resource for remote medical care and advice for expeditions. This activity proved to be very sporadic. One of the interesting actions I became involved with was a claim by a woman who had a ranch in upstate New York who insisted she had an unregistered Przewalski horse, a very primitive horse extinct in the wild but preserved in zoos because thirteen of them had been shipped to the US in the early 1900s. They were bred in captivity, preserving the species from extinction. They are squat, smaller, heavy horses with thick manes and blonde bodies and have a reputed nasty disposition. This woman claimed that her neighbor was an exotic animal importer for many years who had brought animals from central Asia. The neighbor had died and left his horses to her. It was unclear where the horses originated but there was one short, squat but dark brown horse with a thick mane and bad disposition. She thought it was an unregistered Przewalski. I was asked to investigate these claims.

I contacted the woman and arranged for her to get blood samples sent to the Eastern Equine Laboratory at University of Kentucky. The scientists there said they would run a series of karyotypes (genetic evaluations) to determine the horse species of this animal. The upshot is that they ran forty-six different karyotypic tests and the lady had a common horse *Equus caballus*. Basically, she had an ugly, mean-tempered regular horse. She was very unhappy with the scientific conclusion.

A few of the cryptozoology group members also belonged to the prestigious Explorers Club headquartered in New York and asked me to join. I was honored because I had known about the Explorers Club since I was a boy. Prospective members need to have done something in the field of exploration and have two members sponsor them. Among several activities, the one that qualified me for membership was the survey of Philippine coral reefs for the damage caused by dynamite fishing, unfortunately a practice that still occurs. Since we published the report and delivered it to the Philippine Minister of Agriculture, this qualified me to be a Fellow in The Explorers Club. One of my sponsors was the famous shark researcher Dr. Eugenie Clark, who lived near me in Maryland and became a good friend.

This began a fantastic association and opportunities for exploration through The Explorers Club, another defining component of my life. The Explorers Club (TEC) is an approximately 3000-member multidisciplinary, professional society dedicated to the advancement of field research, scientific exploration, and resource conservation. When I first joined in 1992, we received announcements regarding presentations at the Washington Chapter known as the Explorers Club Washington Group (ECWG). After passing on several of the local monthly dinner presentations, I received an announcement of the Explorers Club Annual Dinner (ECAD) which looked quite intriguing. It was to be held at the Waldorf Astoria in New York and the dress was a black tie or native dress, meaning costumes or native clothing from expeditions. There were exotic appetizers and an outstanding speaker list including Susan Sarandon who had just starred in the movie *Gorillas in the Mist* about primatologist Diane Fossey.

My wife and I didn't know anyone in the crowd of 1300, and we proceeded to eat tarantulas on a stick, honey-coated grubs, saddle of beaver, chocolate covered fire ants, grilled iguana, and other strange hors d' oeuvres before we were to progress to the ballroom for dinner and the evening presentations. We could order regular martinis at the bar or an Explorers Martini, the same thing but instead of an olive, the garnish was a sheep's eyeball. The doors were narrow into the ballroom, and I jostled this rather small fellow, excused myself, and introduced myself. He said, "Well hi Mike, good to meet you, I am Thor Heyerdahl." I almost fell over. Here was one of my boyhood heroes and a famous explorer right next to me. Heyerdahl sailed a balsa raft across the Pacific to demonstrate it was possible that earlier peoples could have emigrated to the western hemisphere in ages past from Asia. His fascinating book *Kon Tiki* was required reading in middle school. Never in my wildest dreams did I expect to meet him.

The Explorers Club is headquartered in a historic building on the upper east side of New York city built at the bequest of the Singer sewing machine company heir and donated by famous journalist Lowell Thomas. This five-story edifice is loaded with rare exploration artifacts, photos of explorers, and flags from famous expeditions, like flights to the moon and the descent to the deepest part of the ocean. The board room is decorated with many artifacts and photos donated by Teddy Roosevelt. The heavy table around which I sat for years was the table on which the Panama Canal treaty had been signed. The sled used by Admiral Peary when he became first to arrive at the North Pole is mounted on the wall and the globe used by Thor Heyerdahl to plan his famous balsa raft voyages sits in the upstairs lobby right next to a huge stuffed polar bear. In the Gallery (formerly known as the Trophy Room) is a 15TH century inlaid table from Prince Henry the Navigator and the corner held an ornate glass cabinet that contains several large leather-bound tomes handwritten in French. They turned out to be the official journals of Napoleon's second in command in 1799 during the Egyptian campaign when the Rosetta Stone was discovered. The curator once took me into a small odd-shaped room that had about 60 small leather-bound books handwritten in Spanish and Portuguese that were the actual logs from several 15th and 16th century expeditions. It is an exploration museum much beloved by our members.

Not long after I joined and became active, I had a chance connection to a member of The Explorers Club board and we discussed how the ECWG (the Washington, DC, chapter), the largest of the more than thirty chapters outside New York, could interact to improve the somewhat rocky relations between headquarters and the chapters. There was some friction at that time related to management and finances, but we felt this was mostly miscommunication and misunderstanding. He proposed we have an Explorers Club Board of Directors meeting in Washington followed by a dinner presentation, and I got the agreement from our chapter. The highly successful event reconstituted good feelings between the Washington chapter and the Club headquarters. It did not hurt that we had an outstanding speaker, Dr. Bill Stone, an engineer, and cave explorer extraordinaire. I had invited various media, but the only one who accepted was the science writer for *USA Today*, Tim Friend, and he came as my guest.

This was the beginning of a very interesting friendship in which I was able to take Tim with me to the *Titanic* salvage expedition where he went on a dive to the shipwreck and wrote front page stories about it. Later, I was able to get him on an expedition to Everest and other such activities. Tim, in turn, would use me as a resource for medical issues like prostate cancer and infectious tropical diseases and I was quoted periodically in *USA Today* through Tim or one of his other reporter colleagues. For the expedition to Everest, he was urging me to go and giving me a hard time for not going, with the usual verbal challenges of one's manhood. I told him I do not like cold and do not like heights and Everest obviously was an extreme of both. He told me after he returned that he was freezing in the tent at base camp, he had sleep issues because of the altitude, the wind was flapping the tent so loudly he could not think, he had diarrhea from the water up there, and he was bored out of his mind waiting to ascend to the second camp. He said, "Then I started to curse you for not coming." Some of the best decisions in life are opportunities one turns down.

One day Tim called to invite me to join him at dinner with famous adventure author Clive Cussler who had written several oceanographic exploration stories with his protagonist Dirk Pitt. Tim was doing a feature story on him for *USA Today*. A prolific writer, Clive was a Fellow in The Explorers Club and he had sold millions of books after he started writing novels well into his journalistic career. One of his characteristic signatures is historic sports cars and one was usually prominent in his tales with the back cover adorned with the one specific to the story. I got the idea to borrow my friend Mike Barch's 1956 Mercedes bright red touring convertible to bring Clive from the hotel to the restaurant. He loved it when I pulled up in that car which had been the president of Tanzania's personal vehicle.

We instantly bonded and the three of us had a great time at dinner listening to his stories such as finding one of the very few Confederate submarines ever built, the *CSS H. L. Hunley*, which was lost after she sank a Union warship. Clive invited me to visit him if I was in Arizona where he maintained several vintage cars. I learned that he had over 100 of them stored in the Phoenix area and Telluride, Colorado, and rotated driving these beauties.

As it turned out, a year later, I was a speaker at a cancer conference in Phoenix and called Clive to see if he was available. He suggested I meet him at the Barrett-Jackson auto show and auction that weekend in suburban Scottsdale. I splurged and rented a Porsche convertible for the weekend and would drive the next day to meet Clive.

Clive told me that he would be with his family with a surrey-topped golf cart that I should be able to find in a certain area, so we made plans to meet there. Little did I know the magnitude of the Barrett-Jackson extravaganza with hundreds of thousands in attendance and many more watching on TV. My cute little rented Porsche looked like an old VW beetle compared to the vast array of exotic cars. I could not locate Clive's cart and was about to give up when I finally spotted it. He was delighted to see me when I made it and he said we would walk along with his son to look at the various cars.

I chuckled when I learned that his son was named Dirk. Dirk Pitt is the star of his books. I asked how he selected the surname of Pitt for his protagonist, and he told me he just wanted a short name and it just popped into his mind. We proceeded to survey all the different cars with Clive providing mechanical details on iconic exotic roadsters like Phaetons, Duesenbergs, and J-24 Allards......all of which he owned.

Tim also introduced me to Jay Short, a brilliant PhD researcher, who was president of Diversa Corporation at that time. Diversa Corporation is an industrial biotechnology company that develops high performance enzymes. It extracts microbial DNA directly from collected samples using a proprietary high-throughput process to screen for unique enzymes with potential applications for medicine, biofuel development, environmental protection, food, and other industries. The quest for candidate products sent Jay to exotic and remote places such as the Siberian permafrost, the oceanic hydrothermal vents, Amazonian jungles, and other austere environments. Samples of soil, water, or other components would typically reveal the DNA signatures of around 10,000 organisms, of which 99 percent would be unknown to science. Diversa would then determine what enzymes the genetic material coded for and tested them for their use or effect. Profit from any product was shared with the country of origin. The company has developed products that destroy cellulose and spilled oil slicks. Jay personally has more than 350 patents for his work.

Jay was a perfect candidate for The Explorers Club, and I eagerly sponsored him. After several years and a highly successful initial public offering (IPO), Jay left Diversa to head the E.O Wilson Foundation for a time and then left to start another biotech company to produce conditionally active biologics (CABs). The proprietary CABs developed by BioAtla over the past ten years are very selective antibodies for cancer and are in the mid stages of clinical trials for several tumors with very encouraging results and no appreciable toxicity, a huge advantage. I am on the science advisory board for BioAtla and am quite excited about the potential of these products to make a difference for cancer patients.

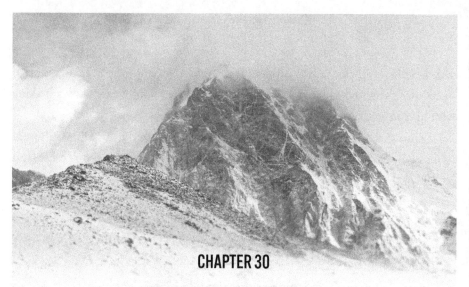

CHAPTER 30

EVEREST AND 9/11

Because of my Explorers Club activity promoting better communication, I was asked to become the chair of the Chapter Relations Committee which got me onto the national scene. I had also been asked to become Vice Chair the Washington chapter with ascension to chair after two years. With national visibility as both chair of the Washington Group and the committee for Chapter Relations, I was drawn into the headquarters politics. A few years later, some board members urged me to run for election to the board. One of them was Dr. Ken Kamler, a hand surgeon who was on Everest waiting to summit when the disaster struck in 1996 and eight climbers died. Ken abandoned his attempt to climb and immediately went to assist the survivors. Although Jon Krakauer's popular book *Into Thin Air* depicts the events, he never left his tent according to eye-witnesses and was not involved directly. Ken, on the other hand, wrote one of the best books about exploration, *Doctor On Everest*, in which he detailed his efforts, particularly with Dr. Beck Weathers, a pathologist and climber who was snow blind and stumbled out of the blizzard when everyone thought he was dead. Beck had sustained very bad frostbite injuries. Beck personally told me he has his life and some of his fingers today because of Ken's efforts. Ken shared his slides with me about the rescue which shows those who survived and their frostbite injuries.

Ken and I remain very good friends and have worked on many projects involving expedition medicine. He wanted me to run for the board but warned me that it would take probably three election cycles to garner enough votes. That had been his experience when he first ran. This is due to an initial lack of name recognition. He was right on the money, and it took three cycles before I was elected. I then spent ten years on the board, a few years appointed at large and then six years as elected. At different times, people wanted me to run for president, but after consideration, I realized that position would require me to spend significant time in New York and I could not do that with a family and relatively small children, not to mention the impact on my professional duties at GWU.

> One of The Explorers Club board meetings was held in Reykjavik, Iceland, at the invitation of President Olafur Ragnar Grimsson. The president was a very gracious host and we held meetings in his spacious house. During one of them, a familiar looking American walked by and waved to us. We realized it was chess grandmaster and world champion Bobby Fischer. He was in trouble with the U.S. government because he had gone to Yugoslavia for a tournament when that country was being sanctioned for political reasons. Fischer fled to Iceland which did not have an extradition policy with the U.S., was granted sanctuary, and lived in the president's house. He later became an Icelandic citizen until his death in 2008.

Everest would continue to interact in my life periodically after that time. During my time as chair of the Washington chapter we got wind of Sir Edmund Hillary coming to Washington to receive the Smithson Award from the Smithsonian Museum, their most prestigious recognition. Sir Edmund was a huge icon of exploration due to his first ascent of Everest and subsequent humanitarian work in the Himalayas to establish schools. He was also the Honorary President of the Club so we contacted him to see if he would be willing to meet with our Washington chapter. We were ecstatic when he accepted, in fact telling his staff to make sure to have time for us. He was a most engaging person and thrilled our group with his appearance and availability. I was invited to a small luncheon with him that included his wife Lady Jane and another Himalayan explorer who created a stunning coffee table book with her photos. He then invited me to sit with his wife at the ceremony in Washington that night where he was to receive the Smithson Award. Sir Edmund regaled the crowd of some 1500 with stories about Everest in a fireside chat format.

Everest was still not done affecting me, however. Sir David Hempleman-Adams is an internationally noted balloonist who was the first to fly a balloon to the North Pole. He was a TEC Fellow in the British chapter of the Club, and he asked me to provide medical care for his planned expedition over Everest. He planned to fly an open gondola over Everest and its height of slightly more than 29,000 feet. This hypoxic atmosphere would be less than one third of sea level oxygen pressure at the Everest peak at the proposed 35,000-foot level needed to transit over the mountain. Furthermore, the temperature at the peak could be as low as -60^0 C and Everest is noted for hurricane force winds. I thought he was crazy to attempt this, but he was dead set (operative word, dead). I told him I could put together a small support team. The plan was for us to meet him on the Tibet side when he landed.

I asked my medical colleague and good friend U.S. Army Colonel Chris Macedonia if he wanted to join me. Chris is an ob-gyn specialist in high-risk maternity but, more importantly, he is also involved with extreme medicine. He became a senior product manager for the Defense Advanced Research Projects Agency (DARPA) which works on very interesting, classified projects, in his case medically related. I brought him to the *Titanic* with me for the salvage expedition and he had been on Everest to the second base camp having gone through the infamous deadly Khumbu Icefall at 18,000 feet. His firsthand experience in this extreme environment would be invaluable.

We assembled the equipment and addressed other issues such as evacuation that we needed to mount a medical expedition to such a climate. Finally, we were ready to go and charted our course to the Himalaya mountains, departing from Washington to New York and then east to the rooftop of the world. I was intending to attend an Explorers Club board meeting in New York on the day before but thunderstorms in Washington cancelled my flight, so I planned to take the shuttle to LaGuardia and connect to departure at Kennedy.

My bag sat on the counter, when suddenly security officers were running through the concourse yelling, "EVERYBODY GET OUT OF THE BUILD-ING!! RUN!" I thought to myself, my God that is a bomb. So, I grabbed my bag which thankfully had not been checked yet and dashed for the pay phone to call my limo driver to return. Who was going to take a cell phone to Everest? This was before widespread coverage anyway. As I called my driver, out of the corner of my eye I saw a low flying plane and then heard a crash. Reagan National Airport was right across from the Pentagon, and this was September 11, 2001.

Horrified, I ran downstairs and out to the arrival area. All cars and taxis had been cleared.... except for one car coming down the road. It was my limo driver. People were yelling for me to take them with me, so I grabbed five of the nearest and sped off. I called GW to see if they needed me as a surgeon. The medical director told me not to come in as there were no survivors though a few victims were transported there before dying. What a tragic day. I can still see that plane hitting the Pentagon.

The expedition was cancelled. There was no way we were going to be allowed to fly over Chinese airspace. Sir David had already shipped his balloon and eventually lost about $1 million on the failed venture. I was now getting the clear message that maybe some higher entity did not want me going to Everest. I got the message, I won't go.

Everest reared its lofty head again for me a bit later when the body of George Mallory was purportedly found. Mallory was a British explorer who took part in the first three British expeditions to in the early 1920s. During the 1924 expedition he and his climbing partner were last seen about 800 feet from the summit but disappeared. There was speculation that he was first to climb Everest before Sir Edmund Hillary in 1953. Mallory's fate was unknown for seventy-five years until his body was discovered on May 1, 1999, by a that had set out to search for the climbers' remains.

The Club was contacted by the explorers who found the body before the public announcement. They wanted an Explorers Club flag to be present and I was on that committee and was contacted by the president for an emergency approval. We award flags to be carried by explorers under stringent conditions. In this case, in consultation with the current president, we would award a special flag. Subsequently the discovery of the body was announced. It remains unknown whether Mallory and his partner reached the summit before they died. The camera he carried was never found though the search for the camera continues.

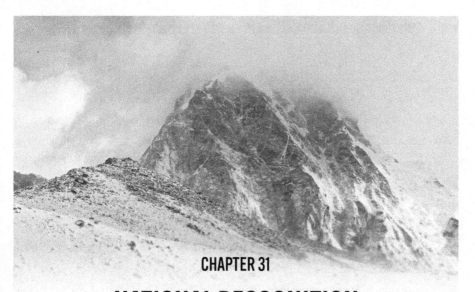

CHAPTER 31

NATIONAL RECOGNITION WITH THE EXPLORERS CLUB

T he Washington chapter of The Explorers Club (ECWG) is the second largest chapter, behind the membership of the New York chapter. With the talent in the Washington area including National Geographic, the Smithsonian, NASA, the World Wildlife Fund, and other such organizations, we have a rich, diverse, and vibrant local chapter. I remember well one evening at a barbecue at my house with several ECWG members when the topic arose about close animal encounters. Each story was progressively more intimate with exotic animals. One guy had been with orangutans in Borneo, and another visited Virunga in Rwanda to observe gorillas. I discussed the very close dangerous encounter with a bull elephant in Africa which stopped within two feet of us. Then Dr. Marty Talbot, a very accomplished wildlife conservationist, spoke up and said that she and her husband Lee had a very close call with a lion.

Dr. Lee Talbot was an icon in animal conservation and widely recognized as author/co-author of the U.S. Endangered Species Act, Marine Mammal Protection Act, CITES, and the World Heritage Convention. A senior environmental advisor to the World Bank and United Nations organizations, he supported ecological research and advised efforts in 134 countries. A global ecologist and geographer, this story took place as they mapped and collected data on animals in Kenya and Lake Tanganyika. The results were the creation of the Serengeti National Park, the Masai Mara National Reserve and much more. He had over 300 publications, many with Marty as an author. Marty said that Lee had killed a charging lion in 1957 in Kenya when they were on that survey. The lion charged out of nowhere into their bush camp. Lee always had his loaded rifle next to him, grabbed it and shot in one motion. The lion skidded dead right at Marty's feet. As we all gasped and had goosebumps, especially seeing Marty's face, I realized again what I loved about The Explorers Club. We had the BEST stories. Lee certainly won that round.

My increasing activity with the Club led me to national committee chairmanships and then to the board of directors where I served for ten years, two full terms of three years each and then as an appointee for different members who left the board for a total of four years. Since I was also chair of the Chapter Relations committee, I was asked to be master of ceremonies one year for the chapter chairs dinner at our annual meeting. This was usually a staid affair catered at the Club with the officers where each chapter chair would give a short synopsis of their chapter events and accomplishments for the previous year.

Since chapters were introduced alphabetically, the Alaska chapter chair was first. I had been warned that Jack Townsend was quite a character known for singing. He did exactly that, singing some show tune in a surprisingly melodic voice, while I shook my head. Really? He must sing to the moose in Alaska.

The next chapter chair from Atlanta started out, "I'm Harry Brooks from Atlanta and I am proud to report that we took sixteen teenagers down into the Amazon....and no one got pregnant." Everybody laughed which continued louder after I said, "Great Harry, thanks, pretty good since your group was all guys." Harry and I have been close friends ever since.

Meanwhile, the Florida chapter chair stood up at his turn and came up toward the podium exclaiming loudly that he was here for his prostate exam and bent over the table. Groan. Well, sometimes you must roll with the punches. I said,

"That is great Hank, but I did not bring my gloves or lube, so you better come to the office like everyone else. Don't worry I will give you a discount." Now the crowd was roaring. It was raucous throughout the whole dinner, and I still have people come up to me and tell me that was the best chapter chair dinner they ever attended. An executive from a large corporation said I should be a professional emcee. I do not know about that but will take the compliment.

Several years later in 2013 I was asked to conduct and moderate the scientific session for the recipients of the Lowell Thomas Awards. This is an annual national Explorers Club event hosted often in New York but occasionally in other cities. Washington was the host that year and the presentations and round table discussions were held at the National Geographic auditorium, a classic beautiful venue.

I was notified that I would receive the Sweeney Award for service to the Club, our second highest medal after The Explorers Medal, a huge honor. Furthermore, it was to be awarded at our annual dinner celebrating

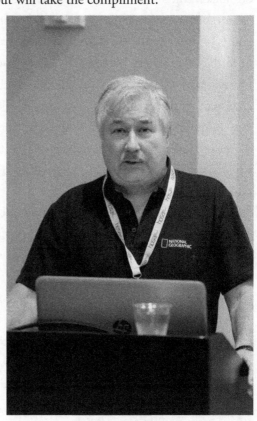

Speaking at National Geographic.

The Explorers Club 100th anniversary. It was a stellar event, and I was seated at the dais next to famous cultural anthropologist and good friend Dr. Wade Davis while on my other side was Dr. Bertrand Piccard, the first man to circumnavigate the earth in a hot air balloon. Next to them was Sir Edmund Hillary, the first to climb Everest, whom I spent a couple of days when he came to Washington to receive the Smithson Award from the Smithsonian. Adventure author Clive Cussler was at the table along with Dr. Kathy Sullivan, the first woman to fly the space shuttle, and Dr. Sylvia Earle, Nat Geo oceanographer Explorer-in-Residence, both longtime friends of mine.

As nearly all the attendees had been ushered to their seats with many still standing, the trumpets blew, and the stirring music began as the president Richard Wiese and the dinner chairman came into the Waldorf ballroom mounted on horses. The horses were skittish with all the noise and people. Richard was led up the stairs astride his mount and they started to bring up the dinner chairman. But halfway up the stairs, the horse reared and threw the dinner chair off onto the stairs where, fortunately, his fall was broken by the people following up the stairs. Chaos ensued. Being a physician, I ran over to the fallen dinner chairman who was all right, so I went back to my place on stage just as the now unmounted horse was led up in front of the head table and faced out on the crowd. Everyone was watching the commotion around the dinner chair, when suddenly, the horse let loose with a big steaming pile right on the head table in front of Sir Edmund and me. We looked at each other and burst out in laughter as the horrified Waldorf staff scrambled out with tablecloths with their eyes bulging in disbelief. It was hysterical! Most of the crowd could not see this fiasco. The old statement about you cannot make this s**t up was literally true here, and I had a front row seat.

As everyone settled down, the dinner proceeded, and medals were awarded. When it came time for my Sweeney medal, the emcee Jim Fowler asked me to step toward the front of the stage to face the crowd. Jim is a famous animal conservationist and celebrity who for years wrestled the alligators and snakes in the background for Mutual of Omaha's Wild Kingdom TV show conducted by Marlin Perkins. Known as Jungle Jim, he was our honorary president, and I knew him well. He was a great raconteur.

Jim started his spiel about the award, and I heard a murmur from the audience that started to increase. Jim had asked me to step to the front of the stage and something was going on behind me. Suddenly, a huge, reticulated python stuck its head through my feet on stage and started to curl around my leg. Of course, I jumped to the crowd's and Jim's delight and laughter. Jim always brought different exotic animals to the Waldorf as a highlight for this dinner, and tropical rainforest eagles circled overhead eyeing the steaks while rare large cats prowled on stage with monkeys chattering from animal trainer shoulder perches. I now have memorable photos of three of us struggling to hold this 20- foot, 150-pound python brute.

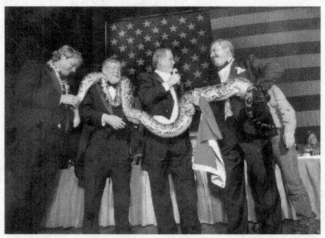

Then president of The Explorers Club Richard Wiese, noted animal conservationist Jim Fowler, and me wrestling with nearly 200-pound reticulated python that Jim let out on stage behind me at the Waldorf Hotel when I received the Sweeney Medal.

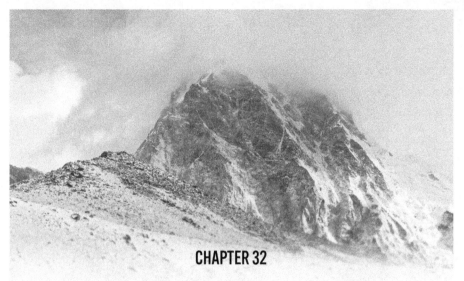

CHAPTER 32

PYGMIES AND AN AFRICAN DINOSAUR

My medical practice sometimes connected me back to my passions. One day in 1996, Bob Ferrante, the general manager of National Public Radio (NPR) radio came in for a routine exam and I recognized his name and voice because he was on the radio frequently. I asked if he would be interested in a story of an unknown animal in central Africa, rumored by some to be a relict dinosaur. He was interested and said that he would connect his science editor/reporter to get in touch with me. Shortly thereafter, Alex Chadwick called, and I instantly recognized his voice. He had created the very popular NPR Radio Expeditions program and did NPRs science reporting. He was quite interested in my story, and he told me that the Anheuser-Busch beverage company was talking about looking into this and was considering mounting an expedition.

We got on the phone with the director of the Anheuser-Busch wildlife productions, John Teichmann, who was heading this effort. After about an hour talking to him about the issues including medical needs, he told me that he had been in touch with others who claimed to know a lot about this animal but that I knew more than any of them. He decided to fly the Busch jet out to Washington to meet with me along with scion Peter Busch, his sister who sat on the board of World Wildlife Fund, radio journalist Alex Chadwick, a dirigible airship engineer friend of mine Ron Hochstetler and a couple others. We hatched the outline of the expedition and began preparations. Because of the remote location and very difficult travel in this triple canopy rainforest, we wanted to explore the use of a small dirigible loaded with imaging instruments to search for large fauna.

A major logistical issue for this expedition was transportation to the Central African Republic (CAR), a chaotic third world country, with significant internal transportation problems. When John and I delved into this, our options to get to the triple canopy rainforest area of interest were limited to either a surface vehicle for an eleven-hour journey (at minimum) over very uncertain roads with questionable security or a small, hired plane with an unknown safety record. Knowing that by far the most common cause of morbidity and mortality in these remote areas is motor vehicle accidents, I was in favor of the three-hour flight, but we had to vet the plane. I called the U.S. State Department for input; we identified a possible plane source and worked with the World Wildlife Fund (WWF), which had a presence in that area, to arrange for a small plane.

Independent of this, an infectious disease physician colleague of mine John Symington contacted me the week before we were to leave, telling me his diplomat brother was coming to town and he had some urological issues he wanted to discuss. The Symington family was replete with diplomats and politicians. I told him I would squeeze him in on Friday but that I was going to a remote area on Sunday for three weeks. If it was not something that needed urgent attention, I could certainly see him. That Friday morning just before lunch, I called the State Department Africa desk which had been working with me to thank them for their assistance. I was very upset at the response that I received that we could not go because there was a situation developing there. When I inquired further about what situation, she told me she could not discuss this now over an open line and would get back to me, but we needed to cancel until further notice. After all these years dreaming about searching for this animal, and the last several months of intense diligence to coordinate our efforts, it was being snatched away from us.

I was utterly dejected when I returned from lunch and the first patient was my colleague's brother Stuart just after arriving from overseas. He thanked me for seeing him on short notice since I was leaving soon. I told him I was not so sure now because there was a "situation," whatever that meant, where I was supposed to go. He said, "Where are you going….to the CAR (the Central African Republic)?" Knowing this was a developing hot zone and probably classified information, I just looked at him and said," Who do YOU work for?" He smiled and said, "State Department" This is often the cover for US intelligence officers, so he clearly was inside that community.

He explained that he was the assistant director of the State Department Africa desk, by amazing coincidence the supervisor of the same people with whom I had been speaking. He explained that the ex-emperor who had been expelled, Bokassa I, was starting a coup to return to power. Jean-Bédel Bokassa was a CAR political and military leader who served as the second president of the CAR until a coup in 1979. He had proclaimed himself Emperor of CAR. Conditions were ripe for civil unrest, the military had not been paid for several months, and he had rallied them to his cause.

Stuart then said that these conflagrations often were very short-lived and blew over quickly. He gave me his cell phone and home numbers and told me he would keep me updated as circumstances developed. In the meantime, I called the capital Bangui to check with the WWF and its perspective of the unrest. The director told me there was a strict curfew, that several people had been shot, and to call before I departed in two days. While I dreaded being caught in deepest Africa in a coup, I was very reluctant to give up on my dream of looking for this animal now that we had progressed so far.

I called the WWF again the next day and was told the situation had stabilized, no one was shot the previous night. This was confirmed by Stuart at State but I should call before I departed the next day. What a dilemma. In the meantime, I had tried to contact John Teichmann, but he was in the south of France at some wine festival with the other guy who would be joining us, Thom Beers, the executive producer for National Geographic Explorer TV series. We were supposed to rendezvous in Paris to leave for the CAR, but they could not be reached. I left urgent messages to contact me to no avail.

I had also not told my wife of these developments. She was off on a college girlfriend reunion, and I did not want her to worry. I also did not want her to try to get me to cancel. I waited until the morning of departure to call WWF again in the capital Bangui and the director said, "The curfew is lifted, no one got shot last night, come on down!" Though I was a bit skeptical, I made a game time decision and left for Paris and the unknown in the jungle.

In Charles de Gaulle airport in Paris, in stumbled the bedraggled duo of Teichmann and Beers. They sobered up quickly when I apprised them of the situation and now, they started to worry, something I had been doing for three days now.

When we landed nine hours later, the city of Bangui was seething, you could feel it in the air. Large groups of people were milling around. The scary scene was mitigated to some degree by the presence on every street corner of the very serious French Foreign Legion, complete with AK-47s and red berets. The WWF was waiting for us and whisked us to their offices immediately upon gathering our luggage. It was here we learned about the logistics of getting to the jungle.

An hour later we were airborne in a small plane flying 2000 feet above a vast rainforest that stretched to the horizon. Our destination was the Dzanga-Sangha Special Reserve which lies in the southwest corner of CAR bordering on Cameroon and Republic of Congo. The 500 million acres together with adjacent reserves comprises the second largest rainforest on earth. It is loaded with megafauna such as forest elephants, lowland gorillas, various antelope species, warthogs, chimpanzees, as well as multitudes of bird and insect species. Large numbers of hippos and huge Nile crocs patrolled the river while we ate our meals suspended twenty feet above the riverbank. This is the area that renowned National Geographic biologist Michael Fay walked through in his famous megatransect a few years later.

I had been in touch with Michael Fay before we departed while he was back briefly in the US. He is a biologist who has dedicated himself to animal and land conservation and spent seventeen years in the area. He had lived in the jungle in a small lean-to hut for a while deep in the reserve, studying the animals, particularly elephants. We had determined that we would be thirty kilometers apart though in different countries (he in the adjacent Republic of Congo). Transportation was so difficult we would not be able to connect there. In discussions with him, he knew of the legend of the animal we sought but told us there were two versions, one with a long neck like a sauropod and another with a short neck, point on its nose, and a fierce demeanor. He said the latter was most likely an occasional errant black rhino, known for its aggressive disposition, which wandered into the rainforest from its usual savanna habitat and really scared the local pygmies. He felt this was the basis of the legend. Frankly, it made sense, though we hoped to learn more about these rare appearances.

Down in the jungle area, the locals did not care or even know about the impending coup. In fact, the coup waned shortly after it had started. Bokassa had a trial in absentia and was sentenced to death. He returned to the CAR in 1986 and was put on trial for treason and murder. In 1987, he was cleared of charges of cannibalism, but found guilty of the murder of schoolchildren and other crimes. The death sentence was later commuted to life in solitary confinement, but he was freed in 1993 and died in November 1996, shortly after our expedition and his aborted coup.

We landed on a dirt airstrip that we had to buzz first to get animals off the runway. Met by a Bantu ranger, we stowed our gear and immediately left with him to view elephants in an area set up by noted researcher Andrea Turkalo, who was studying the pachyderms form of communication. Elephants emit sounds that humans cannot hear, and it was fascinating to learn about this currently well-known form of animal communication. We had to walk twenty minutes through this impenetrable jungle to a clearing (called a bai) where an observation stand had been erected. These infrequent clearings are created by elephants and this huge one contained some elephants, several species of antelope, warthogs, buffalo, birds of many types, and literally millions of butterflies. An idyllic creek meandered through the middle of the clearing. This was the Garden of Eden and utterly fascinating.

Shortly after we started toward the bai, the Bantu ranger stopped and instructed us in broken English, "If you see gorilla, look down. If you see elephant, stop. If you see buffalo...run like h** l", and we chuckled. His perceived joke on us turned to reality when minutes into the trail, an elephant walked right across our path ten feet ahead. You could not see or hear it until it was right in front of you. We paid attention.

Our lodgings were quite comfortable though we were sure to securely tuck our mosquito nets around us to discourage the huge huntsman spiders in every room. Huntsman spiders do not nest but wander around hunting and supposedly have a "wingspan" of about eight inches. I have a photo of one in our room where one of our "roommates" legs extended beyond either side of a 7-inch board, so it had to have a wingspan nearly a foot. They are also called rain spiders because they come inside when it rains. Well guess what, we were in a rain forest, it rained daily! These huge spiders were always with us.

Tasty dinners were served in a stilted open hut suspended above the Sangha River loaded with flotillas of hippos and huge Nile crocodiles. Days were spent reconnoitering the jungle or hunting with the indigenous pygmies with their crossbows and poison arrows for their dinner.

The Bay'aka pygmies lived in small igloos but foraged constantly as true hunter-gatherers. They were very generous with their community meager rations though we deferred. They are delightful friendly people, frequently singing melodically and did not care about the political situation or coup.

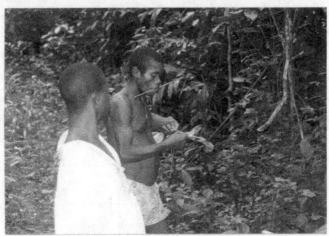

Pygmies making poisonous arrows for hunting.

One night John and I stayed in the small hut previously occupied by National Geographic explorer-in-residence Michael Fay while he observed the forest elephants. It was small, and we left the door open to get some air because it was very hot and steamy. Here we were, a couple of city boys deep in the jungle.

We decided to sleep with our boots on and fully dressed in case we had to move quickly. All night long we lay awake listening to animals, some of them large, moving around us in this tiny lean-to. We also heard a loud animal scream which sounded like it was next to us but was probably at least a half mile distant. I was told later that poachers were likely hunting an elephant, very sad indeed.

Just before dawn, though we could barely hear them, several elephants walked within a few feet of us to go to their wallow about 100 meters away. Mike Fay warned us we might have to shoo elephants off our paltry front porch. This wallow was quite interesting in that the elephants used their tusks to loosen and then ingest the clay. It turns out the clay contained kaolin and was likely used by the elephants to soothe their upset gastrointestinal tracts. Kaolin is one half of the active ingredient of Kao-pectate, a widely used medicine for upset stomachs in humans. It was very interesting to see this behavior, it is a gauge for elephant intelligence in my mind. I was thrilled to sneak quietly down toward the wallow, stopping 50 meters away to observe the elephants up close.

We were made aware of an American who had come to the CAR jungle to record the pygmy music. This guy had adapted to life there, taking a pygmy wife who was half of his 6-foot 4-inch height. Louie Sarno turned out to be from New Jersey and very jaundiced from a recent bout of hepatitis. He was quite overjoyed to see us, and we took him to dinner at the only restaurant in the tiny provincial town of Bayanga. It turned out that dinner was fish and we truly wondered at the origin of our entre as we sat by the open riverside window watching all the debris and dead fish float by us. Well, as I have always said, if you have a good sauce and it is cooked through, I am not sure I need to know the species of the dinner special. Fortunately, none of us got sick despite the polluted river water occasionally splashing on us.

Upon return to Bangui, we went out on the town with German mercenaries we had met who had run guns for Ugandan rebels against Idi Amin. One stop was an exotic bar right out of Star Wars with exotic-looking Somali waitresses, CAR bartenders, and Dutch, Italian, and African patrons flavored with Cape Verde music. I left them all about midnight, knowing full well how this was going to end but I had to meet the American ambassador early the next morning. Sure enough, those guys got in about 5 a.m. not entirely sober despite skinny dipping in the hotel pool with some expat talent. My meeting with the American ambassador that morning was punctuated by her exclamation that she was glad we made it because the small plane we had flown had gone down three times in the past year.

The return trip was marred by a shakedown at the airport customs where John had to pay $600 to get out and he barely made it aboard. He had bought a few small displays of the beautiful butterflies and was accused of smuggling. I had bought only one and was spared for unclear reasons except I had nothing valuable and most of my money in my shoe.

Sadly, the elephant researchers and other scientists also have had to flee persecution. We can only hope the fascinating bais and rainforest are not too violated.

It was truly difficult to transform back into a medical practice after such a spectacular road trip! And I get a Pavlovian response when I get a call from John Teichmann, I start looking for my bush hat and passport.

As a sequel to this adventure, I was invited a few years later to a special National Geographic event where Alex Chadwick was going to host Michael Fay and recreate the CAR environment with all its sounds on the auditorium stage. Alex is a master at sound integration and the pitched tent on stage with surrounding sounds of the jungle brought it all back for me. Alex announced to the crowd that he was nervous because there was one person in the crowd who had been to this very remote area, and he hoped he had it right. He was referring to me. It was perfect! I had a strong déjà vu of being in that rain forest. Afterward, I stood back as many people crowded around Michael Fay and Alex. Mike was now famous for his megatransect of the rainforest, a feat the pygmies even thought was crazy. When Mike Fay was told that Dr. Mike Manyak was here to see him, he parted the crowd and rushed over to me, giving me a big hug. We had not met previously but he remembered our conversations and knew that I had stayed in the hut he had stayed in, way off the beaten path. Everybody in the crowd wondered who I was.

One other funny story about Mike Fay and Alex Chadwick is illustrative of Mike's unique character. Mike would periodically come back to the US, often to Washington, and he would stay in the office of Gil Grosvenor, former President of the National Geographic Society, and editor of National Geographic Magazine. It had a shower, and he did not need a hotel, and he got around mostly by bicycle.

Mike is very used to living off the grid. One time he came back and decided to camp in Rock Creek Park which is a large national park that bisects Washington DC and goes from Maryland to right next to the White House. This is not open to the public for camping, but it is not very well policed for such activity and there are some homeless people who reside in the park. Alex decided to stay overnight one night and interview Mike Fay in his tent. His stories were fabulous. What a couple of characters! They both have been dinner guests at my house, and we were most entertained exchanging stories. Isn't that what life is all about? Who has the best stories!

Mike nearly died about five years later when he was gored by a bull forest elephant. He survived because the elephant's tusks passed on either side of his chest while he was lying on the ground (luckily, he is thin) and only damaging soft tissue which healed. I am told he has now returned to Gabon where he is helping the government to stop illegal fishing. He is now trying to establish a marine protected area, a result of having worked with another fellow National Geographic Explorer-In-Residence who is the head of the Pristine Seas program, Enric Sala. I have enjoyed several detailed conversations with these elite explorers.

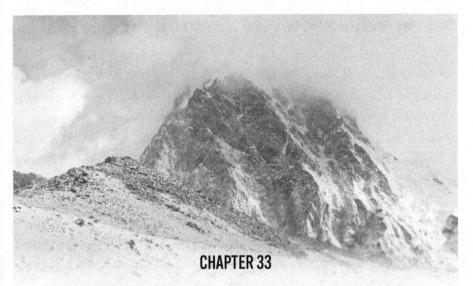

CHAPTER 33

DIVING FOR MONGOLIAN ARTIFACTS

B ack in The Explorers Club breakfast line at our annual national meeting, the very accomplished diver and explorer friend Peter Hess introduced me to Steve Schwankert, the founder of the first scuba dive shop in China. Steve lived in Beijing. After I was introduced, they said, "Hey, do you want to go to Mongolia?" I said, "Sure. What are we going to do?" The reply came back, "We are planning the first scientific dive in Mongolia." This is the kind of conversation you got into at the Club. They needed medical coverage. Naturally, I replied, "H**l yes", and another expedition was hatched.

Scuba diving in Mongolia? Wait a minute, isn't that a landlocked country in the middle of Asia with the Gobi Desert covering a significant part of it? Yes, but a large lake on the northern border adjacent to Siberia offered just such an opportunity.

Siberia? Isn't that really cold? Yes indeed, again, but the lure of the first exploration of this body of water proved very attractive.

Lake Khovsgol (pronounced HUHVS-gull), not far from its better-known Siberian neighbor Lake Baikal, is the second largest lake in Central Asia. It holds almost 70 percent of Mongolia's fresh water and 0.4 percent of all the fresh water in the world. Revered by Mongolians as sacred and surrounded by mountains in a protected Mongolian national park, this narrow, 80-mile-long body of water resides at an altitude of 5000 feet and looks like one of the northern U.S. Great Lakes. The lake is frozen more than it is fluid and therefore constitutes a challenge requiring a dry suit and dive table calculation for altitude.

The objectives of the first scientific dive in Mongolia were to determine the quality of the lake water and to evaluate the nine known species of fish. Rumors of a large unknown fish referred to as an "underwater deer" did indeed raise some concerns, but we were equipped with side-scan sonar to aid in identification of any such submerged strangers. The exciting opportunity to identify new species overrode any misgivings. Furthermore, there were Russian shipwrecks and about forty cars and trucks that fell through the ice in addition to rumors of Buddhist relics thrown by monks into the lake during a time of Russian persecution in the 1930s.

Getting to Mongolia itself was quite a hike for our expedition with about a dozen Explorers Club members. Long flights brought us to Beijing and then to the capital Ulaan Bataar where about 1.4 million of the 2.9 million Mongolians live. This largely undeveloped city was undergoing change due to the influx of money from foreign mining interests. After a night to gather our equipment and relax at the Genghis Khan bar, we flew three hours to the regional city of Moron where we boarded land rovers for the twelve-hour trek to Lake Khovsgol over very poor roads but beautiful vast, open steppes. There was humorous speculation about how the inhabitants referred to themselves, whether it was Moronians or just Morons. This was just an observation and in no way impugned their intelligence or character.

Arriving beaten up by the rough roads, we stashed our gear into our gers. These octagonal reinforced tents with cots, also known by the Turkish name yurt, were actually very comfortable, especially with the fire going inside, necessary because temperatures fluctuated from 80 degrees in daytime to 30 degrees at night.

Diving in remote Lake Khovsgol was very challenging. There were no dive centers, no air fills, no compressors, and certainly no palm-frond covered cabanas serving post-dive piña coladas. The nearest dive center was five hours by flight, so we had to bring everything including back up gear. Our expedition moved over one ton of equipment, including sixteen air tanks, two air compressors, and personal gear for ten divers. We hoped there wouldn't be hyperbaric problems because the nearest hyperbaric chamber was located several hours flight away and was essentially unavailable from a practical standpoint.

Dive planning and safety briefing occurred in the morning before entering the water. Some of us patrolled the lake surface with sonar while others dove, with a watcher on shore for safety given the diving conditions. The water proved to be quite clear (and cold with sharp thermal gradients), and water samples demonstrated no biological or chemical pollutants. Dive planning was complicated because of the cold and the 5000-foot lake elevation, circumstances that had to be figured into dive tables. Furthermore, dives were with dry suits, a two-layered somewhat cumbersome but suitably warmer dive suit. We located a few interesting Russian era shipwrecks but no Buddhist relics or gold items as had been rumored. The lake was full of a large cod-like species and the smaller Siberian grayling that were unafraid of humans since there is little tradition of eating fish and low human population. We could swim right up to schools of these fish without spooking them. It certainly was tempting to snag a few to throw on the grill but we respected our hosts and refrained. We did not see any taimen, the largest trout in the world. with a record length of 7 feet and weighing 230 pounds. They are primarily found in rivers. Maybe that is the "underwater deer".

My return to the airport was highlighted by my Mongolian driver who drove as fast as he could over terrible roads. He spoke no English and I knew no Mongolian, so we communicated by hand signals and grunts. Trying to get him to stop for a biological break with hand signals without being misinterpreted is a story for another day.

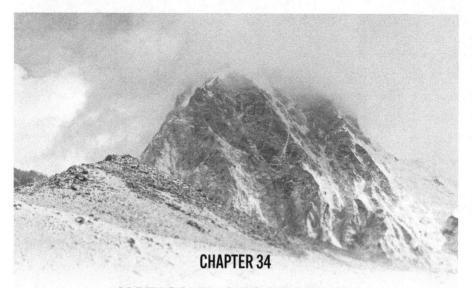

CHAPTER 34

NATIONAL GEOGRAPHIC
AND EXPEDITION MEDICINE

O ver the years, I began to work with National Geographic on issues related to expedition medicine. Before this, I was co-editor on a major textbook, *Expedition and Wilderness Medicine* which I edited with two others. I wrote the chapter on medical evacuation. The book is now considered a major resource for expedition medicine.

As an offshoot of the book, we editors decided to conduct a medical conference on expedition medicine. One of the attendees was the nurse practitioner who ran the Nat Geo medical office, Karen Barry. She told me they had a doctor, but he had no expedition or tropical medical experience. She had to prepare all the Nat Geo explorers for remote medical problems, vaccinations, and outfit them with medical supplies. She said sometimes she had some unusual issues and did not know who to call. I told her to call me anytime for anything and I would be glad to assist her. Thus began a very good friendship and we still communicate regularly.

Karen was not kidding about unusual issues. One day after the conference she called and said a photographer on a shoot in Indonesia had a problem. He had been filming Komodo dragons, the largest existing lizard which could grow to almost ten feet in length and weigh up to 150 pounds. These monsters feed mostly on carrion but are opportunistic feeders. Their mouths are loaded with many types of bacteria in addition to saliva that has venom and an anticoagulant. A feeding strategy is to bite potential prey, especially if large, and then follow them while they get sick and weaken. Their photographer had gotten close, and a dragon had spit in his eye.

Karen had done the correct thing to have the patient's eyes copiously irrigated and I instructed her not to patch the eye to allow any exudate to drain and to start him on oral antibiotics. I further advised that if the eye reddened or he developed a fever, he needed to be evacuated to save his eyesight. Fortunately, he did not need to be evacuated.

> The title *Lizard Bites & Street Riots* for my second book came from a story about Komodo dragon saliva spit into the eye of a Nat Geo photographer. The book was selected by USA Today Best Books Awards as well as the International Book Awards as a top five finalist for best travel guides and essays in 2016.

Another time, Karen called and asked how to get antivenin for puff adders. Puff adders are quite venomous and particularly dangerous because they are well camouflaged and can be found close to urban areas. She told me she had a group in Mali in Africa filming elephants. An off-season cyclone had struck causing flooding which combined with tremors from stampeding elephants had flushed a huge number of snakes out into the open. I told her to contact the Pasteur Institute in Paris since this was in a previous French colony which maintained relationships with its former colonial power. I also told her to zip up the tents and keep everyone inside, something she had already done. She was able to locate puff adder antivenin at the Institute and fortunately no one was bitten.

Karen called again with a question about one of the Nat Geo writers deep in the Amazon who had a complaint of abdominal pain. I got on the phone with him and ascertained that he also had a bulge near his umbilicus. Being suspicious of an abdominal hernia with potential to become strangulated leading to bowel obstruction and perforation, I told him he needed to return home and I would arrange for him to see a good surgeon at GWU to evaluate the need for surgery. The surgeon phoned to tell me I made a good call about an impending intestinal strangulation and that the writer was on the surgical schedule to repair his hernia before it could become strangulated.

One of the more interesting calls from Karen at Nat Geo involved artists going into the ancient sewers of Paris, purportedly the largest sewer system in the world. It appeared that nearly three levels down in those sewers, some very interesting artwork from centuries ago had been discovered, much like graffiti in our tunnels and sewers in more modern times. The French government would not let any researchers into the sewers without a vaccination for leptospirosis, a bacterial disease which is passed in urine of rats and many other mammals. I had experience with treating this disease in the Philippines where every time there was a monsoon flood there would be an ensuing outbreak in the poor communities affected which can result in fever, muscle pain, bleeding from the lungs, meningitis, and kidney failure. Again, we went to the Pasteur Institute, and they had vaccines though the characteristics of this disease challenged immunologists to develop an effective safe vaccine. Nonetheless, we were able to obtain the vaccine and permits. About six months later, the fascinating colorful artistic results of this urban expedition graced the cover of the National Geographic Magazine.

A few years ago, Karen contacted me to get some assistance with a Nat Geo expedition headed by internationally recognized film producer Steve Elkins. The group had discovered a huge unknown pre-Colombian city buried in the jungles of Honduras. Their discovery was documented in the NY Times #1 best seller *Lost City of the Monkey God* by Douglas Preston. One problem they had encountered in the fetid, humid jungles were the omnipresent millions of sandflies. These sandflies transmitted a nasty parasitic disease, leishmaniasis, through their bites. It was nearly impossible to avoid bites in this environment. This is a difficult disease to treat, and it requires restricted medications. Forty percent of the group contracted the disease and were under treatment at the NIH ICU because side effects of the drugs used were very bad. I told Karen I knew about this disease and the victims were in about as good a place as they could be. Leishmaniasis is a very disfiguring disease which presents one of three ways: a cutaneous form with extensive skin deformities much like leprosy; a mucocutaneous form with ulcers of the skin, mouth, and nose, again like leprosy; and a visceral form which starts as skin ulcers but then goes to the liver and spleen which can kill the victim.

Steve Elkins was a speaker for the recent workshop run by the New York Council of the Boy Scouts at The Explorers Club headquarters to qualify scouts for the Exploration merit badge which I had created. He told me there were about a hundred scouts there and he wanted me to know that the booklet I wrote about exploration to accompany the merit badge had absolutely captured the essence of exploration as well as anything he had ever read. This was quite a compliment!

The physician who covered Nat Geo was retiring and they had been talking to me for three years about becoming the next doctor there. There were some problems however, which in the end could not be surmounted. One was that the pay was quite low. The previous doctor had worked for significantly less than the market rate for such a position and Nat Geo was reluctant to pay more. Secondly, and more importantly, Nat Geo was undergoing major changes. It was eventually purchased by the Disney Corporation and many corporate changes were implemented. It is still in a state of flux but at least the decision was made to keep the medical office and not outsource health care.

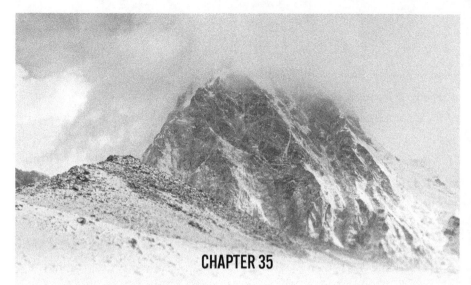

CHAPTER 35

HIGH THREAT SECURITY NETWORK AND CHIEF MEDICAL OFFICER FOR TRIPLE CANOPY SPECIAL FORCES

cott Harrison introduced me to a high threat security company, Triple Canopy, which provided protection to embassies and personnel, often in troubled areas in the world. Scott had retired from the CIA and created his own risk management and security company and consulted on security issues for Triple Canopy. Triple Canopy was founded by Special Forces under highly decorated US Army Colonel (ret) Lee Van Arsdale and had 7000 contractors deployed in Iraq, Afghanistan, and southern Israel. They were looking for a chief medical officer.

Shortly after the footprint expedition in Tanzania, I began as chief medical officer at Triple Canopy. My duties at Triple Canopy included coordination of all medical issues with senior staff and their deployed employees. I had sixty-two medical personnel reporting to me from battle zones. One item of business was to overhaul their medical formulary. Employees were deployed for three months at a time in stressful combat circumstances. Mostly interested in their physiques and condition, a fair number of them liked to use enhancing substances they discovered on the internet. The problem was that these were often various forms of anabolic steroids with unwanted side effects and essentially banned by the US State Department which provided the large security contracts. The government does not want contractors to be driving armored vehicles and using automatic weapons while under the influence of these types of compounds which can cause personality changes such as rage.

After furlough and now returning to duty they had to pass a drug screen. If they tested positive for steroids, they were out of work. I am sure some were not aware that these supposedly muscle-building compounds were forbidden steroids. We did have a few that tried to game the system. Two of them came in and said that they were under a doctor's care for testosterone injections for hypogonadal (low functioning) testes. Hypogonadal testes are a medical controversy because some men with supposedly low levels function just fine and do not exhibit signs of low testosterone. The problem for the returning contractors who were trying to use these products was that I am a urologist and know all about this. If you give standard testosterone supplements, you will not get supraphysiologic levels of testosterone (above the normal range). If you took anabolic steroids, you most certainly will.

I told everyone that if they had supraphysiological elevated testosterone, they would be disqualified for work. One of the men in question provided the name of the doctor who was injecting him. It turned out to be a female gynecologist who was advertising that she would provide testosterone injections for men, a highly suspect practice. I called her and she immediately hung up quickly when I explained I was CMO for a U.S. State Department sponsored company and a urologist and what she was doing was dishonest and likely illegal. Fortunately, this was an isolated incident, and we did not have any more trouble with steroids.

There were some very different problems encountered on this job where medical personnel reported to me from battle zones. Problems were often mundane such as a broken ankle playing touch football but there were also serious injuries and death from mortar rounds and high velocity projectiles. We scrambled to get proper medical care on site and arranged for evacuation when stable which was an interesting exercise when conducted in three different languages. One time I received a call from a forward-operating base (FOB) on the very dangerous Pakistani border. One of our men had a fever that had spiked and was given what sounded like an appropriate broad-spectrum antibiotic. He had dropped his fever for a couple of days but now it was back again, and it spiked like that every day or two. I did not like the sound of that and asked if he had been tested for TB which can present like that, a perplexing recurrent fever. They evacuated him and got him tested and he had TB disseminated throughout his body. I saw a lot of TB in medical school, and something rang a bell for me. Fortunately, he got appropriate therapy. The same old story repeated often in diagnostic situations, if you do not think about a disease, you cannot consider it.

TB was the source of another problem I encountered. One of the men on furlough received a notice from the state of Florida nearly three months after he was rotated out and scheduled to return. The notice said he was likely exposed to active TB on his return flight from Abu Dhabi and needed testing and a chest x-ray. When he contacted us at headquarters, I found out that we had thirteen employees on that Delta airlines flight, that there had been a passenger who deplaned and was taken to the hospital in Atlanta with a high fever and cough and was diagnosed with active TB. None of the other employees had been contacted.

I then attempted to speak with Delta management to determine where the patient had sat, knowing that anyone within two rows was at higher risk from exposure. These passengers would require testing and x-rays and further monitoring. I was completely stone-walled by Delta, they would not put me in touch with their CMO either. I did not need to know the gender, nationality, or any other personal identifying information except the seat in which that person had sat. I was very unhappy with this response from Delta and asked which news media they would like me to tell this story. The Triple Canopy attorney refused to back me up because the company did not want it known that Triple Canopy personnel were traveling by commercial aircraft, a potential political issue. Consequently, we had to test all thirteen employees periodically for a year in addition to having all the men have chest x-rays.

Another issue was sleeping disorders, often due to stress. We had several requests to use zolpidem (known as Ambien), but the problem was that it can have residual effects, so it wasn't advisable for the users to use it while on duty using automatic weapons or driving armored personnel carriers. We ended up modifying slightly the regulations of the U.S. Air Force who does have similar issues for pilots.

I was asked to attend the weekly meeting with the Department of State security team about status in the areas where the men were deployed. State was spending hundreds of millions of dollars on these programs and monitored events closely. These contracts went out for bid to security companies like Triple Canopy. The State security folks were delighted to have a doctor present as an integral part of the team since medical issues came up regularly. This meeting was where we resolved the sleep disorder issue. Another major issue was that the medical personnel on the ground could not get enough strong pain medication. These are controlled substances, often opiates, and State was rightfully concerned about theft on the other end, a real potential issue. The downside of that is that the men who needed it for injuries sustained fighting could not get what was needed. I was an advocate for the men and wrangled with State Department officials about this. Finally, we came to a compromise, and I got some concession but not to the desired level.

Triple Canopy wanted me to do a site visit of their training facilities outside of Baton Rouge, Louisiana, which was a large compound used jointly by the Louisiana state police. They sent me with their head of recruiting Bill Culpepper, former Sergeant Major of the Army, the highest non-commissioned officer in the U.S. Army who had been in the presidential detail. Rather laconic at first, he opened up over the several days we were there and told some great stories. One involved an Iraqi detachment that wanted to board the empty presidential plane on the tarmac late one afternoon. No outside weapons were allowed on the plane for obvious reasons. When the lead guy with an automatic weapon sneered and said he was coming on board, Bill just turned to me and calmly said," I had to break his arm". In his mid-50s now, Bill was still formidable at 6 feet 4 inches, about 240 pounds of muscle. He is EXACTLY the wrong guy to mess with and the guy I would choose to be at my back if an altercation broke out somewhere. That story still makes me chuckle.

So does the story Bill told about being with a few senators and their wives on a fact-finding mission in a southern Italian city at a restaurant with dignitaries that included the chief of police. Bill went to get flowers for the ladies from a vendor outside of the restaurant. When he reached to pull out his wallet, the vendor pulled a knife out and tried to rob Bill. I asked Bill what he did, and he turned to me laconically and said, "I had to break his arm." The commotion caused by the now howling vendor brought some of their party outside including the police chief. The would-be thief was screaming that he was calling the police when the police chief roared, "I AM the police!" and his police colleagues drawn to the scene promptly dragged this guy off to jail.

During my site visit to Baton Rouge, I met several times with the training director who happened to be an 18 Delta, which is a Special Forces medical sergeant. These guys are excellent battlefield emergency medical technologists and he and I got along famously. We went through their protocols and meds. They put me through some of the training courses which included defensive driving and escaping hostage situations. They taught me how to drive from the passenger seat when the driver had been shot, quite interesting for this old ambulance jockey. They taught me how to do a 180 degree turn which is quite difficult even if used in the movies and unless you have the right type of car, it will drop the transmission. Stability of transmission and power is why they always used Ford Crown Victoria models. The training instructors had me practice shooting with their M 240 machine guns, incredibly powerful guns with an effective firing range up to 1800 meters.

The leaders of Triple Canopy thought it might be useful for me to go to Iraq to the Green Zone to observe the medical facilities and protocols. My wife was not amused by this, and I was a bit apprehensive as well. They reassured me that I would be in full battle gear in an armored convoy from the airport and that I would always have a security detail with me. However, the conflict significantly escalated in Iraq at that time and all non-essential personnel were being evacuated. Triple Canopy decided to have me stand down. I always have wondered what being in a real battle zone was like.

Although I didn't end up working full-time for Triple Canopy, I remain in touch with some of the senior management as they have moved into other positions. Jeff Denton, the former senior VP of Operations and Green Beret paratrooper, designs fascinating high-tech arms for our soldiers. Decorated marksman and former VP of Operations and Army Ranger helicopter pilot Jay Christy heads security for a large bank corporation.

I was now in the tent with security and subsequently consulted with other corporations for medical health and security. Accenture had nearly 500,000 employees at that time, and I was asked to become the Chief Medical Advisor for Crisis Response, providing expertise to the security team for their hundreds of daily traveling employees all over the globe. My duties consisted of interfacing with the bio-surveillance program and presenting a quarterly review of exotic or dangerous diseases in addition to sporadic emergency responses. Therefore, we were prepared and had discussed Ebola before the African outbreak that scared the world. We also identified the Covid-19 virus as dangerous in November 2019, at the beginning of the pandemic based on a small report of some deaths in China from an unknown respiratory virus. That report was expunged from the internet by China, but it certainly raised our suspicions.

We continue to worry about one of the deadly flus which do not often infect humans acquiring the ability to attach to the human respiratory tract easily. Bird flu and swine flu are in that category as is MERS, Middle East Respiratory Syndrome, which is a coronavirus. SARS is another bad one, a coronavirus which somehow had been contained in China before it escaped, but that was lucky.

Accenture wanted to increase our security knowledge and experience and sent me to IJet, a high threat security company created by former NSA senior analyst and radiation physicist Bruce McIndoe. He had a training exercise for a couple of days that included didactic instruction and field tradecraft. We learned how to identify and react to a kidnapping attempt and then had to respond to a random simulation the next day while at a restaurant. Then we were taken to the nearby mall and after instruction in countersurveillance had to identify characters in the crowd of shoppers who were surveilling us as we split up to cover the whole mall. It was an interesting exercise and even the seasoned security personnel could not spot them.

In Washington, a group of us would gather regularly after work. This included various security specialists such as the International Money Fund (IMF) Director of Security, British intelligence agents, CIA station chiefs, and NSA senior personnel. One common thread was that all were friends of Scott Harrison. The reason I was included was because of my work as chief medical officer at the high threat security company Triple Canopy.

I became close friends with several of these guys. Warren Young is a highly decorated former Australian Special Forces officer who had an MBA. The natural intersection of health and security was key for him with over 600 IMF personnel traveling daily and personal responsibility for the IMF Managing Director. In fact, I was with Warren the night he received the call about the arrest of the Managing Director Dominique Strauss-Kahn (known as DSK) in New York. DSK is a French economist and politician who attained notoriety due to his involvement in several sexual scandals. He was originally backed by French president Nicolas Sarkozy. Rumors that DSK was going to run for president of France were controversial and then DSK resigned in the wake of an allegation that he had sexually assaulted a NYC hotel maid. The sordid details included the presence of his DNA which he could not deny and there was strong feeling within the intelligence community that DSK was set up by the Sarkozy camp. DSK's natural tendencies for promiscuity certainly lent itself to this theory and his potential candidacy was sabotaged.

Warren's Swiss wife also had some stories she shared when at my home for Thanksgiving. She had been the personal airline attendant on the private plane of Democratic Republic of the Congo dictator Joseph Mobutu who was smuggling conflict diamonds to Geneva. She carried the diamonds and was watched closely. Very interesting work.

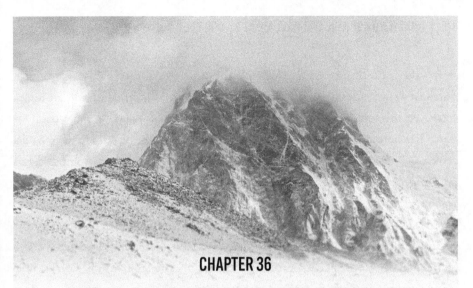

CHAPTER 36

MEDICAL CARE OF EXOTIC SPECIES

I was occasionally consulted about urological problems of exotic species. The Washington Zoo would sometimes call with questions. During my time at the NCI, the veterinarian with whom I worked quite a bit called me because their very expensive boar hog had blood in his urine. This animal was in a long-term study about cardiovascular disease and a great deal of money had been invested in his health. Therefore, they did not want to lose this animal to a disease. The vet asked me to operate on this huge animal, a hairy 450-pound beast with big tusks. I told her we should approach this as a human problem and get as much imaging information as we could first, then decide if an open procedure was indicated. Since the blood could come from anywhere from the kidneys to the bladder and external genitalia, the less invasive information we could acquire would benefit all of us, including the hog.

We were able to get a limited x-ray study of the upper urinary tracts that showed prompt filling of the kidneys with contrast and rapid excretion, telling us there was no obstruction and no obvious tumors in the kidneys and ureters which are the long tubes that propel urine from the kidneys to the bladder. The next step is to evaluate the bladder with a small telescope, not a small feat in this large animal. Fortunately, we were able to improvise with a pediatric scope used to evaluate lungs. However, the foreskin of the hog is attached to his belly unlike human counterparts. Furthermore, the urethra, the tube that leads from the bladder to the outside, took a 180 degree turn back into the bladder, again different from humans. I was able to negotiate the telescope into the bladder and rule out presence of a bladder tumor. Hogs do not generally have large or obstructing prostates, and this was confirmed to be the case here, again ruling out a potential source of bleeding that occurs in human males. In evaluating the foreskin, it was noted to be abraded and an injury here was the likely source of bleeding. The correction for this was a simple circumcision by making a slit in the foreskin with no need to excise tissue but rather just suture the edges to themselves to stop any bleeding. This cured the problem, and the vet was ecstatic that I had saved the hog from a huge operation. Who else among my colleagues has done a circumcision on a boar hog?

A good friend of mine, Dr. Steven Seager, a veterinarian at the National Rehabilitation Hospital, also happened to be a pioneer in insemination of endangered species. He was a developer of electroejaculation which is exactly as it sounds. This technique had been developed for spinal cord injury patients. Steve had been at the forefront of employing this procedure on exotic animals. He had the most amazing photos of exotic animals he had worked with including orcas, orangutans, snow leopards and all the other big cats, and even a hornbill bird. Some of these specimens represented the first-time semen had been collected from this exotic Noah's Ark menagerie.

Steve asked me to go to the Berlin Zoo to help him extract semen from both the white rhino (for the first time ever) and the highly endangered black rhino (the second time ever). We arrived in Berlin in the early evening and went straight to dinner. After a good repast and some tasty German beer, Steve suggested we go to the Berlin Zoo where he had a key to enter at night. It was very weird opening the zoo with no one there in the dark. As we walked around on the zoo paths, it was quite eerie because the animals all knew we were there and could see us a lot better than we could see them. It felt something like the movie *Night At The Smithsonian*.

The next day we caught up early with the zoo vets. The first order of business is to sedate the white rhino. How does one sedate a triceratops? You must dart them in their cage. As I was taking photos of the rhino through a small, barred window in the cage, I suddenly realized the rhino's horn was much larger in the view finder. He had charged the window and thrust his horn through that window, missing me by six inches as I jumped back, and I got a great photo of the ceiling. Quite a thrill!

Rhinos can be 4000 pounds of pure muscle with a thick leathery hide. There is nothing soft on them. The reason the rhino had to be electoejaculated was that the twenty-five-year-old had developed arthritis in his knees so he could no longer mount the cow from behind. These are such expensive animals and endangered, so it was felt that artificial insemination was a good approach.

Once the rhino was darted, the dicey part started. You must give enough anesthesia so you do not get in a cage with an irritated behemoth but not too much to over-sedate them because you could kill a million-dollar animal. Rhinos sedated tend to be like humans drinking alcohol, when they get groggy, they lean on the wall. We could not have that happen because if the rhino slides down the wall, we would not be able to move the legs and reposition the animal to work. Now there is a bit of a dance that occurs, and someone has to go into the cage and get the rhino's attention, much like dancing in front of a bull to get them to charge. Then once the now wobbly animal comes away from the wall as the anesthesia starts to take effect, the assistants must be there with bales of straw to place under the animal as it falls to avoid breaking its leg. Despite the intricacy of this process, the vets did a stellar job, and we now had the animal in the middle of the floor, giving us access to the body parts we needed.

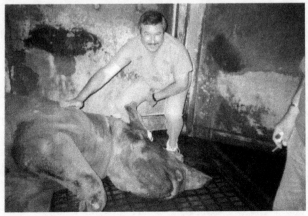

Caption for rhino photo here

The rhino had to be cooled off, so a hose was constantly in use keeping its temperature down. Next the ultrasound probe was placed in the rectum. For humans, the probe has a 6-centimeter bulb at the end which scans the prostate. In this case, Steve had designed customized probes for all the exotic animals and the one for the rhino looked like a rocket-propelled grenade attached to a broomstick. Picture a football on a stick. I declined the opportunity to palpate the rhino prostate, primarily because we had surgical scrubs with a short-sleeved shirt and standard sized gloves. That means my entire arm from the edge of the glove to the edge of the shirt sleeve would be buried in rhino excrement.

> Ultrasound images of the rhino prostate showed it to be relatively small compared to the rest of the body dimensions and it doesn't grow circumferentially around the urethra, like in humans, so rhinos do not get urinary obstruction from prostate growth.

Once the probe was properly positioned, the rhino received a small electrical jolt to cause ejaculation. To extract the semen required milking his organ to get the semen into a beaker. The vet called for his graduate assistants and three young women appeared to do this. The rhino penis was about three feet long and as thick as my arm. The tip of the organ has four flanges which helps the rhino maintain position during insemination so he would not slip out of the female. I could not help but think what a great adaptation, I could probably use something like that. As the graduate students milked the semen toward the end of its organ to collect the fluid, I could not help but wonder how they explained to others what they did that day at work.

We were now rewarded with a beaker nearly filled with semen. We ran to the microscope and put a sample on a slide to look for sperm viability and normal shapes. The sample was teeming with active, viable sperm that were nearly all normal in shape and functionally swimming. The head vet was very happy. I was told this was the first time this had ever been accomplished in the world. The sample was immediately taken by other vets and placed on ice in a travel case, and they departed shortly thereafter for the Vienna Zoo where the vets there were waiting to inseminate their female rhino. I understand that I am now an "uncle" for a twenty-year old rhino in that zoo.

Once the white rhino procedure was completed, we then performed the same process on the black rhino which is much more highly endangered with only about 4000 black rhinos left, mostly in the Mkuze Game Reserve in northern South Africa. I have visited there and was quite anxious being on foot looking for the notoriously short-tempered black rhinos. The black rhino is a bit smaller than the white rhino, but the same precautions and processes were used for the procedure and with the same positive results. That was the second time in the world that a black rhino had that procedure.

Steve Seager asked me six months later to go with him to Belfast, Northern Ireland, to work on gorillas at the Belfast Zoo. A bonus was that the Belfast Zoo also wanted us to evaluate a highly endangered feline, the African Golden Cat, a rare thirty-pound animal that looked like the North American cougar.

The story in Belfast was that a lowland female gorilla which had a one-year-old male baby was poached in Mozambique fifteen years earlier. After being kept captive in a cage for a year, the young gorilla was sold to a third party before the Belfast Zoo officials got word of it and purchased it for the zoo. Although it had been seen copulating, there had been no pregnancies and zoo officials were worried that it was infertile. This would be a real shame because a wild caught gorilla would be able to add to the very limited gene pool to help preservation of the species. They contacted Steve to evaluate the gorilla and try to get a semen sample.

We flew to Belfast and stayed at Steve's idyllic ancestral home for a day and headed to the zoo to evaluate this 400-pound animal. The gorilla in question was sequestered in the vet area. What was eerie was that the other gorillas congregated just on the other side of the wooden slat fence and could be seen looking through the cracks between slats. They certainly seemed to know something of significance was going to occur to one of theirs. It was unnerving to look at them observing me so close to them.

Back in the vet enclosures, we prepared for surgery which entailed doing a testicular biopsy in addition to semen extraction. As this huge gorilla began the anesthesia induction process, I noted that the anesthesiologist was having some trouble trying to place the endotracheal tube to administer the inhalational anesthesia and oxygen. He told me when asked that he was not sure about the tube location which would be critical to make sure both lungs were insufflated. In humans, we can listen to either side with a stethoscope and can hear breath sounds in that respective lung. However, in these huge barrel-chested gorillas, it was not possible. The anesthesiologist asked me if I would like to try to intubate, a skill we learn on both the ambulance and from my surgical training. I moved to the head of the table where the gorilla was sedated. He had a large oral cavity, as you can imagine, and large sharp canine teeth. I was able to visualize the vocal cords which is your landmark to go between and taped the endotracheal tube in place after placement. It appeared that there was equal insufflation in both lungs, and we proceeded with the procedure. It was a unique thrill it was to intubate one of these precious animals!

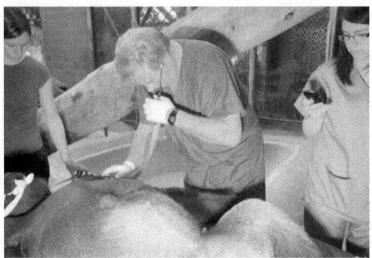

The huge barrel-shaped chest of an adult gorilla makes placing the tube for anesthesia challenging.

Gorilla male genitalia are surprisingly small in comparison to human counterparts. In fact, human males have one of the largest ratios of genitalia size to body size. The electroejaculation process was not very successful because we only extracted a small amount of fluid with no sperm detected. Therefore, we proceeded to a testicular biopsy which was successful in obtaining the proper tissue that contained spermatic tubules. The surgical wound healed without complication. This is important because animals can scratch or bite an incision, causing infection or dehiscence of the wound. Two weeks later we learned that the spermatogenic tissue was not normal, so it was felt that the animal was indeed sterile.

One year later, despite that interpretation, the Belfast Zoo sent me photos of a baby gorilla and told me another female was pregnant, both by our patient! We suspected that the spermatogenic tissue may not have matured at the time of the biopsy.

We moved on to work with the Asian Golden Cat, a polymorphic colored, medium-sized cat with a head-to-body length up to three and a half feet with a tail up to two feet. It weighs about thirty pounds, about three times the size of a domestic cat. DNA analysis reveals this cat species diverged from a common ancestor up to 8 million years ago and this rarely seen endangered cat is now found in the northeastern Indian subcontinent, Southeast Asia, and China.

The Belfast Zoo wanted to breed their male and female specimens. The problem is that the larger male is characteristically very aggressive and is prone to kill their female counterparts in addition to mating with them.

The zoo decided to house them in cages that ran parallel to each other in the hope that they would acclimate to each other. The male cat and smaller female had been caged next to each other for a year and seemed to be relatively relaxed around each other. Before risking death of this rare female cat, the zoo wanted to know the male sperm quality before putting them together.

The cat was anesthetized and intubated, and Steve proceeded to electroejaculate the animal and collect the semen. The probe was substantially smaller than the rhino probe and even the human counterpart. I still wonder what size the probe was for the hornbill bird. When we examined the specimen microscopically, we were all quite pleased to see millions of viable sperm swimming normally. The vets were ecstatic because now they could put them together, and if the female survived, she might be pregnant.

Another time I dealt with exotic species was when I was the guest of my friend Dr. Laurie Marker, the highly decorated founder of The Cheetah Conservation Fund (CCF). CCF is a research and lobby institution concerned with the study and sustenance of the country's population, the largest and healthiest in the world. Laurie had created a fascinating, highly successful, self-sustaining conservation area and recently opened a guest house for tourists on site at the time of my visit in 2018. The over 35,000 square kilometers of her reserve has over 50 cheetahs, many of which she had reintroduced to the wild after salvaging them from poaching. She has an infirmary on site to deal with ailing cheetahs and happened to have one in kidney failure when I was there. I was able to help start intravenous fluid replacement which is easier than with humans because you can place the needle and catheter under the skin but not in a vein to transfuse fluids because they are absorbed. In addition, Laurie has a sophisticated and very valuable genetics lab with genotyping of all her cheetahs and a genetic tissue bank for all kinds of animals. We were able to add to that tissue bank when I was there when we came upon a caracal which sustained a mortal injury from a car just before we arrived. We took some tissue samples from the beautiful cat as it was taking its final breaths, but sadly we had no chance to save it.

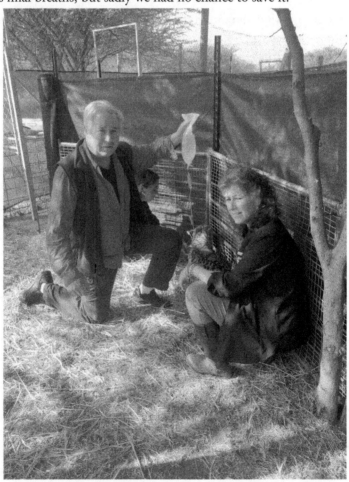

Treating a cheetah in renal failure with Cheetah Foundation Director Dr. Laurie Marker.

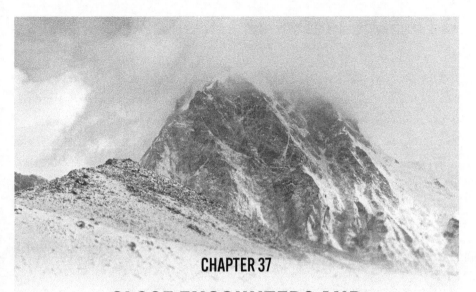

CHAPTER 37

CLOSE ENCOUNTERS AND AN AFRICAN BUSINESS PROPOSITION

R hinos had appeared in my life periodically, usually by choice but occasion-ally a bit unexpected. Having seen them up close, I have a very healthy respect for bumping into them on their own turf. I was on a rhino walk with a South African game ranger quietly observing a female and her adolescent offspring from about 100 meters away when some noise spooked mama. She turned and charged up the trail right at us. The ranger jumped out waving his arms and yelling and the rhino and son veered off the path thirty feet from us. They were incredibly fast! The ranger explained that they have poor eyesight but have great hearing and smell (which I knew) and she did not know we were there initially.

On that same adventure, once we had settled down after the surprise charge, the big male started coming slowly over the hill towards us, 150 meters away at the time. The rhinos were familiar with this area because the rangers put out hay to feed them while they sheltered at night in a protected area with stalls open on either end for rapid egress. The ranger had us put a large tree between us and the advancing rhino which was curious about us. We circled the tree as he continued to come closer, it was now about 30 meters away. The ranger then said, "Time to go" and we backtracked slowly toward our Range Rover. The rhino suddenly stopped as five African elephants came around the corner 100 meters away in single file, coming to eat. The rhino stopped following us and stood still. It was explained to me that one of the elephants did not like the rhino and they had confronted each other before. The rhino was a monster, but these elephants dwarfed him. From my perspective on the ground, it was a most awesome sight.

Another time when I was with my wife in Africa, we went for a rhino walk tracking a white rhino with a game ranger and Zulu guide. We followed a healthy distance behind as the ranger explained that the rhino could turn at any time and charge and that we had better pick out a tree to climb. I said to my wife that we are not shopping, and you better grab the first tree you can scramble up and move fast. Shortly thereafter, one of us stepped on a twig that snapped and the rhino wheeled around quickly. We slowly eased back, never taking our eyes off this huge animal. Fortunately, it did not charge but I guarantee you the adrenaline was flowing.

Black rhinos are quite endangered with only about 4000 still around, 2500 of which are in the Mkuzu Reserve in South Africa which I visited. We went on a rhino walk here as well. Our Zulu guide had been all but comatose through most of the trips we had taken with him but on this one, he was on full alert.

Black rhinos are known to charge without provocation and to arrive in a bad mood. As we walked through the brush, me watching for snakes and him watching for rhinos, we came upon a family of white rhinos grazing about 100 feet away across a small stream. We walked very carefully by this prehistoric scenario and had no trouble, but these giants were aware of us. Our Zulu guide was much more alert when we were in the bush though because of his fear of the black rhinos.

Another elephant encounter occurred when I was staying at Phinda in South Africa, this time with my wife. I was on an invited speaking engagement for the South African Urological Society, and she came as we planned to visit a game reserve as a side trip. We had our own game ranger assigned to us. We had seen a lot of animals including big cats up close. The small plane we flew in from

Johannesburg had to buzz the runway twice to shoo rhinos and giraffes off the dirt landing strip. It was an idyllic place, newly opened, and part of the Conservation Corporation Africa (CCA) conglomerate which had thirty-eight game reserves in six southern African countries. The organization was dedicated to having wildlife corridors for animals to move more easily and the CCA CEO Dave Varty was well known and the owner of Londolozi game reserve, famous for big cats. CCA itself was bankrolled by the Getty family and Tara Getty had a gorgeous place right on the reserve.

On one game drive, our game ranger asked what we would like to see that day. We had not seen a lot of elephants and he knew where there was a rather large herd we could observe. The herd turned out to be in an area that had to be approached down a narrow one lane path surrounded on either side by very thick bamboo. We stayed well back from the herd on that lane. I turned around and then noticed a large young bull elephant coming down the road behind us.

I poked the ranger and pointed, and he said, "Oh no, nobody move" as he loaded and cocked his high-powered rifle. There was nowhere to go for either us or the elephant that continued to advance. We thought it might stop but it continued almost to our land rover and started to lower its head to butt our vehicle. The ranger yelled and the elephant stopped as the ranger hissed in a low voice to us not to move a muscle. This huge beast then slowly walked and squeezed to the side of our vehicle and stopped right next to my wife and just looked at us from two feet away. Barely able to breathe, I noticed my wife starting to scoot slowly toward me and I whispered to her to stop moving. After what seemed like an eternity but was probably five minutes, the elephant slowly passed on and we could breathe again. The ranger, visibly a bit rattled now, moved, and lowered his rifle.

This experience led to a very fascinating thread in my life. I had a very enlightening conversation with the head of HR for CCA before we departed for home. I asked her who covered their medical problems and found out that they had little coverage. I told her I could put together a team to do this and CCA was interested. I went home and assembled some good friends to go on a site visit to determine what we could do. Two key people were an infectious disease specialist from Harvard and a dentist, my old friend Kevin O'Keefe who had gone on to do a lot of charity dental work in remote Himalayan areas.

When we arrived in Africa at Phinda with our small team, we had a boisterous dinner at the game reserve with Tara Getty and some of the CCA folks. Joining our table was another guest whom we did not know but was welcome. He was a young Belgian businessman and was a bit in awe of being with the doctors. Kevin, never one to miss an opportunity, told him he could make him a dentist the next day as his assistant. The local tom-toms had broadcast that a dentist was in the camp, a rarer event than even having a doctor there. Consequently, there were fifty villagers lined up when we got up in the morning. Kevin dressed the Belgian in a mask and gloves and had him pass instruments to him. One catch was that he had few instruments and basically could only pull a diseased tooth or leave the patient alone. Since these teeth were very painful for the patient, they did not mind having the diseased tooth pulled. The Belgian was ecstatic to be an assistant, a source of mirth for the rest of us. They spent the day pulling teeth and the thankful villagers praised the dentist. There was one problem, they could not pronounce his last name, O'Keefe, so they called him Doctor No Teeth. The Zulus had a good sense of humor. Sometimes life is funnier than fiction.

On that same trip, we had to be careful on the trail going from our cabanas to the main dining area because big cats and even rhinos came through there on occasion. We walked down the trail constantly looking furtively over our shoulders. On the path I jumped back with great alarm when our infectious disease doc yelled and jumped back pointing to the grass. Thinking he had seen a mamba or other bad actor, I was amazed to find out he was pointing to a tick on the end of a grass frond. Ticks carry a lot of bad diseases, but they don't attack you. We laughed loudly and he took a lot of grief warning us of an impending tick attack. It still amuses me and makes me smile thinking of that tick event but somewhere, infectious disease expert Peter Hotez is frowning thinking about making light of tick diseases.

I had one of my best game drives ever leaving Londolozi to go to the Zulu village to meet with the Zulu chiefs and village elders to discuss their medical needs. We saw an elephant in the road in front of us that we had to wait to move off, we had hyenas eating a kill about ten feet from us just off the road, and we startled a group of impala, one of which was speared by a lion waiting in ambush right in front of us.

The meeting with the tribal elders and chiefs was engrossing. It was no surprise to find out that they most coveted primary care but did need some specialty care for obstetrics and pediatrics. We could set this up for them, but the issue would be longer term funding.

In the meantime, the CCA general manager Les Carlisle pulled me aside and said that if we did not have support with a revenue stream, it would be short-lived no matter the best of intentions. He tasked me to come up with a business plan that we could present to its board of directors. I then huddled up with my infectious disease friend and we kicked around various ideas.

What we presented was ingenious according to the CCA CEO. Basically, any visitor to the 38 CCA game reserves had to carry their own travel medical and evacuation insurance and CCA offered various products from third parties. Since I had been involved with evacuations and worked with a very good company as a consultant, we figured out for a nominal sum tacked on to the already very expensive travel package, we could provide such services including trip cancellation, lost luggage, and other benefits like return of remains, a difficult and legal challenge in the event of a fatal adverse event. Travel companies and destinations like game reserves do not like to advertise these benefits to avoid any perception of danger, but some danger certainly exists. For example, far and away the most dangerous problem was a motor vehicle accident which may be unlikely in the game reserve but would be much more prevalent in the cities through which travelers traversed. The extra fee would be split between our company and CCA. Some of this money would go toward building and funding clinics in the villages surrounding the game reserves. CCA believed that if services were provided to such villages, the inhabitants would be very favorable to CCA and not poach animals. This suggestion seemed to be a win for all parties with an income stream for both CCA and us and services for the villages.

When we presented this to the board, the concept was well received. We were told that CCA would get back to us. The CEO Dave Varty then flew to the U.S. to meet with me about further details about implementation. When we had hashed out the details, he said he loved the idea and would take it to the board. If this worked, I would have to go to Africa a few times a year to check on things in one of my favorite locales. This could be a dream come true.

Unfortunately, when Dave returned, he found the board had drastically changed and he was ousted as CEO. The board declined to follow through on our plan for insurance coverage.

A few years later when I was on the board of directors of The Explorers Club, the president asked me if I would help him review curricula vitae of applicants for executive director. He sent me ten resumes and one of which was from someone from CCA. The delightful young woman who had helped with our presentation had applied. I told the president I knew her and would strongly recommend her. She subsequently became the executive director and ended up marrying the president who was a TV personality.

In another strange coincidence a few years later, I ran into Les Carlisle, the CCA general manager in New York. I was on The Explorers Club board and was asked to retrieve our awardees at their hotel for a big gala, the Lowell Thomas Awards. The theme that year was animal conservation and The Explorers Club awarded a corporation in recognition for contributions to exploration. CCA had been chosen. With great glee I found out upon my arrival at the hotel that Les Carlisle was the CCA representative. We had a lot of laughs including the story about when I was at Londolozi and a highly venomous green mamba came boogeying through the middle of the dining area and everybody dropped everything and scattered. They are fast and aggressive.

The other very distinguished awardees who squeezed into the limo with me were equally fascinating, such as the famous biologist Dr. E. O. Wilson, prolific author and ant expert from Harvard. He made me smile when he simply introduced himself as Ed. Equally self-effacing and humble was famous zoologist and big cat expert Dr. Alan Rabinowitz, executive director of the Science and Exploration Division for the and head of the Bronx Zoo. The evening was topped off when I escorted actress Stephanie Powers to the dinner and stage. She had been highly active in African animal conservation for many years along with her now deceased husband, actor William Holden.

As you can see and I was warned, Africa can really get under your skin. The idea of a travel medical coverage product and company still resonated with me after the CCA deal fell through. I was invited by National Geographic to a special dinner in recognition of Dr. Jane Goodall, the famous primate researcher.

When I asked at our table who covered the medical aspects of the Nat Geo explorers and family, Bill Allen, the editor of the magazine said they did not have coverage. I then launched into my story of the CCA business plan for medical and evacuation coverage and told him we could do the same for the 8 million Nat Geo subscribers as a member benefit for a small fee. He was intrigued by the idea, and he contacted me a few days later to discuss this in detail. After much discussion the senior management decided not to pursue my program because profit margins were very tight on the magazine and any added cost would make the profits precarious. In coordination with the nurse practitioner Karen Barry who ran the Nat Geo medical office, however, we were able to arrange to have medical evacuation coverage for staff and explorers through Global Rescue, a very competent medical evacuation company. Little did I know then that I would work periodically with Karen on some of the most bizarre medical problems faced by Nat Geo and me.

Jane Goodall's presentation was highly entertaining, and people lined up to speak to her afterwards. Scott Harrison had told me he knew her rather well because he was her next-door neighbor in Tanzania when he was CIA station chief there. He told me to say hello if I ever had an opportunity to meet her. I patiently waited in line for others and when it was my turn, I said, "Hi Dr. Goodall, my closest friend said to be sure and say hi to you. Scott Harrison." She stared at me and said, "Scott?? How is the dear man?" Apparently, they had libations as neighbors on regular occasions. She made me sit down with her and tell me what Scott and I were doing and then she said, "Come with me young man!" She proceeded to grab my hand and march me across the stage like a schoolteacher in front of everybody to meet the director of her institute. I felt like a little kid. Remembering this encounter makes me smile every time I see her on a show or TV special.

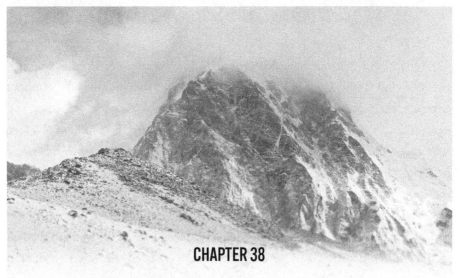

CHAPTER 38

CAREER CHANGE: BIOTECH

Times were changing in medicine, and I concluded that it was time to move on from this position after 10 years as chair of the department. Since I had many relationships in industry and had worked on numerous products, I chose this route. I was offered a vice president job for a relatively small biotech, Cytogen Corporation, that used small radioactive particles attached to very specific proteins called monoclonal antibodies to image prostate cancer. I had worked with this company and was lead author on the pivotal study taken to the FDA for approval. Now they were interested in having me work full time, so I pulled the trigger and left GWU.

Working in industry requires adjustment from the academic milieu and though the company wants your academic approach, it must be within the confines of the corporate focus, and budget. I was a primary driver of their physician educational program which was necessary because of the complex nature of the product. I reanalyzed existing data from some investigators to provide clinical outcomes that demonstrated the value of the product. Although it seemed like I was a prophet crying in the wilderness (and maybe a crazy one at that) and this work was often dismissed, some key scientist/physicians began to listen. Fifteen years later, I have been justified as this system is one of the hottest topics in prostate cancer management. I have had some gratification from former colleagues who have contacted me to say that I was right about this imaging system.

One time at Cytogen we brought in a consultant. At dinner we ordered oysters and asked her to take the last one remaining. As she bit into it, something crunched, and she pulled an object from her mouth. Thinking it was a piece of shell, we were all truly amazed when she brandished a pearl from her hand about the size of a pea. None of us nor the restaurant staff had ever experienced this. Though it was a bit irregular, it was clearly a pearl. The odds of finding a natural pearl in an oyster are 1 in 10,000 and 1 in a million for finding one of gemstone quality. The average value of these very rare dinner plate pearls ranges from $200 to $400.

Cytogen Corporation suffered the throes of a small biotech with chronic underfunding of projects. The company became a target for acquisition and was acquired by another slightly larger biotech. The problem was that they shifted focus to another product we had unrelated to prostate cancer. Thus, it was time for me to move on after four and a half years. Being in a small biotech had and I had learned a lot about corporate medicine and now looked for something more substantial.

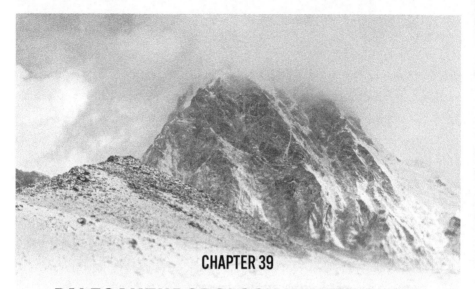

CHAPTER 39

PALEOANTHROPOLOGY IN KENYA AND MORE DANGEROUS ANIMAL ENCOUNTERS

I n the interim between leaving GW while I was consulting, my exploration activities continued, and I was fortunate to have some unique experiences. Again, Africa was the backdrop for excavation of early human artifacts in Kenya with Dr. Rick Potts, one of the most pre-eminent paleoanthropologists in the world who is Director of the Smithsonian Human Origins Program as well as chair of the Smithsonian Anthropology Department.

In 2006, Rick invited my family and I to Kenya to the site of their highly productive early human fossil and artifact excavation on the edge of the Rift Valley in an area famous for such fossils. Well, Rachel refused to go when she heard there were bugs. Susanna was literally getting back from her three-week Australian trip and rightfully said she would be exhausted. My wife said she would like to go but no way was she going to let two teenage daughters stay home alone, a recipe for disaster. Of course, fourteen-year-old son Tim was game. Tim and I left for Kenya.

When we arrived in Nairobi, we checked into the hotel and left for dinner at the Carnivore, a famous restaurant like a Brazilian churrascaria where skewers of meat are brought to the table and portions carved off. The Carnivore fare was camel, crocodile, impala, eland, duiker, warthog, and Nile perch with various local fruits and vegetables. It was unique and delicious, and Tim still raves about that dinner. The next day we left with Rick for the dig site. He had tents set up for us, but it did not take Tim long to come to my tent and ask if he could sleep there because he was worried about hyenas and snakes. There was plenty of room and I was delighted to have him join me as we gazed at the millions of stars visible. Trips to the bathroom were nonetheless undertaken with flashlight and boots on.

In the daytime, I marveled because these world class scientists such as noted Smithsonian geologist Dr. Kay Behrensmeyer would take Tim by the hand and say, for instance, "Today I am going to teach you geology" or some other scientific aspect. However, they also put Tim to work; he was under the jurisdiction of Dr. Briana Pobiner as they excavated, bagged, and labeled one million-year-old human artifacts for further cataloguing. One day, paleoanthropologist Jenny Clark (Rick's wife) took Tim to go see a baboon colony up close. At the end of the day, the scientists would go over the relevance of that day's discoveries at the dinner table with sundowner cocktails, a very educational experience.

Tim and I said farewell to our scientist friends after a week and headed through the Masai Mara and into the Serengeti. We paused to watch animals for a couple of days. There were large herds of migrating ungulates trailed by predators. We even saw a large Nile crocodile take down a wildebeest just like in the National Geographic films. We then moved on to southern Tanzania to three different small private camps for more game viewing in a large area known as the Selous, named for a famous game hunter who donated the land. This area had only opened for game visits fifteen years earlier and was relatively undiscovered by tourists.

At our favorite small camp, we became friends with the camp manager and were assigned a Maasai ranger as our game driver. She warned us that we needed an askari (guard) to accompany us up the path from our very comfortable accommodations as dusk began. A Maasai warrior with a lion spear (and a high-powered rifle slung over his shoulder) walked with us to the dining area. Not five minutes later, the manager came in and asked us if we had just come up the trail before her. When we told her yes, she said let me show you something. There were paw prints of a large leopard on top of our footprints indicating that he followed us up the trail.

After dinner we retired for the evening, I was awakened at 4 a.m. by a deep guttural growl sounding like T Rex in Jurassic Park very close to our upscale tent. I tried to wake Tim quietly so he could hear but it was not repeated. I am sure that would have made the hairs on his neck stand up. Clearly that big leopard was still around.

The next morning our driver got us up at dawn, telling us the lions were moving and we should go see the activity. You could hear them roaring and they were close. We scrambled into our clothes and hopped in the jeep. Our driver explained that an adolescent male had come on the territory of the alpha male in the area. The alpha male was not happy and was basically frog-marching the teenager off his property. The teenager, true to human form, was dragging his feet and taking his time, aggravating the adult.

After a while, the lions veered off into the savannah and stopped. Our driver pulled up parallel to them. Suddenly, the big male adult looked at us and immediately charged from 50 meters away. Our driver yelled, "Hang on!" and floored the jeep. That lion gave us quite a jolt and got within 20 meters within a few seconds. When we finally stopped, I asked our driver if the lion would have stopped. "Maybe" he grinned in response. I had never seen this behavior from lions. Tim got a great photo of the lion as it started its charge.

I was able to talk our Maasai driver into telling us how he became a man in his village. Basically, as a 14-year-old, he had to hunt and kill a lion on foot with a spear and he told us the whole story but only after I told him Tim was 14 years old and I wanted Tim to hear what our driver had to experience. It was fascinating.

The next day we moved on to a camp in another area of the Selous. There was a lazy small river meandering through the property and our new driver said we could look for leopards in the trees lining the river. In the distance a mile away was a small herd of elephants browsing in the grass near the river. We slowly proceeded along the riverside but suddenly were interrupted by a disturbance in the brush behind us and an elephant abruptly charged us, gaining rapidly on our jeep. Once again, we heard our driver yell, "Hang on!" This was no faux charge like I have witnessed previously. This elephant was angrily trumpeting with ears laid back and trunk out straight as she raced toward us. She got within 20 meters of us. It took a mile for that elephant to drop off the chase even though we pulled away from her. The driver speculated that the elephant group had an experience with poachers which explained the unannounced real charge.

We then headed back home through the Tanzanian capitol Dar es Salaam with another truly exciting road trip under our belt. This was one of my favorites because I shared it with Tim. We had been charged by a lion, charged by an elephant, and dug one million-year-old early human artifacts.

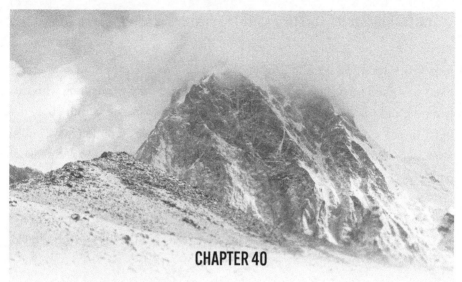

CHAPTER 40

THE DEEPEST CANYON IN THE WORLD

A nother great expedition occurred when close friend and explorer Piotr Chmie-linski asked me to join his group to Colca Canyon in southern Peru. I met Piotr years earlier when he approached me about joining the Explorers Club.

I inquired if he had any field experience and he replied without pretense, "Well, I kayaked the length of the Amazon, and then I interrupted him, "Excuse me, did you say you kayaked the length of the Amazon???". I just started laughing and said, "I don't think we are going to have any trouble getting you into the Club. I will be happy to sponsor you."

Piotr knew about my expedition medicine experience and wanted me to be the medical officer on the return to Colca Canyon with the Polish explorers who first publicized this area. It became a tourist attraction for Peru that has brought significant money into the area. He intended to take thirty-three people ranging in age from sixteen to seventy into very rough country starting around 13,000 feet high up in the Andes. We went over all the protocols, medications and supplies, and the medical histories of all expedition members. We made sure that everyone carried medical evacuation insurance. Only one member claimed he had his own medical evacuation insurance already, and I had him verify he was covered. The rest took out a short-term policy with Global Rescue (GR). I sat down with the GR CEO Dan Richards and his VP of Operations to plot out any evacuation route if needed from deep in the Andes. The company had classified information about small airstrips throughout South America that we could use in an emergency.

Once we rendezvoused in Arequipa, the nearest city of any size to our destination, we left in a caravan of mules and on foot. I started out on a mule but a few hours later, the mule must have sensed he had an inexperienced gringo on his back because he threw me off. Thank God it was against the mountain instead of the unguarded other side which went down over a mile. That was enough to cure me of riding and, swearing in Spanish, I fell in line with the other explorers on foot. My marching companion, a photographer for the Chicago Tribune, is a great guy and we marched together the rest of the day.

This expedition scared me because of safety issues. The trail was quite treacherous and so narrow at times that you had to turn sideways and put your hand on the mountain as you shuffled along one foot at a time on this six-inch-wide ledge. You couldn't put your full weight on your lead foot because every so often your foot would come loose and the mass of small stones (known as scree) for your foothold would give way. I asked the Peruvian guide with me if mules or people ever fell off the mountain and he smiled as he said, "Sometimes."

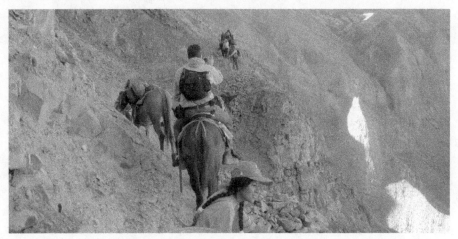

The trail down the Colca Canyon was quite treacherous where one stumble could mean serious injury or death.

As we came single file into our first camp, the only flat place in the entire journey because indigenous people had created terraces for planting crops, the vista was an aerial view like that of a plane landing, but we were walking. As I got to the campsite, exhausted, I heard a yell and turned just in time to see a member of our team rolling rapidly down the mountain. He had gone fifty feet and was stopped by running into a large patch of cactus. As I jumped up to yell, 'Don't move him!" the first Peruvian guides got there and promptly stood him up. I was concerned about a serious injury to the spinal cord, fractures, neck, and head injury and that's why a victim should not be moved until evaluated and stabilized. They laid him down so I could evaluate the damage.

Examining the victim, I saw he had bad lacerations of his hand such that the tendons were visible. There were no apparent fractures, but he could certainly have non-displaced fractures of the vertebrae from the neck down. He could move all his extremities. He was alert and oriented with no apparent skull deformities or blood from his ears. His abdomen was soft indicating no likely internal hemorrhage at least at this time. He had many cactus spines in his body which were painful. I told him we had to evacuate him because the lacerations needed evaluation for tendon injuries and suturing. He was also at risk for infection, something potentially fatal in a remote area although we had oral antibiotics.

The victim turned out to be the only one of us who had medical evacuation coverage with another company, Medjet. Contacting them was not easy and our satellite phone coverage was limited to short windows when the necessary satellite triangulation needed for connection could occur at 9000 feet in the Andes. I finally got through, explained the situation, gave my credentials, and told them they needed to evacuate him because he could not climb or ride a mule back to the top and going forward was not an option. Medjet then said he did not have medical evacuation coverage, only medical transportation, meaning that if I could get him to a hospital facility, they would come to get him. The victim was certainly not aware of this distinction. I told the medical director that if I could get him to a medical facility, I did not need them. He needed evacuation.

The company essentially said it could not come to get him, abandoning him in his predicament. I brought the bad news to the suffering victim still in a lot of pain. I explained that he absolutely needed evacuation and I was a consultant with a company that had prepared for this trip. I contacted Global Rescue and they said they would have a helicopter ready within fifteen minutes when I gave the word to execute our prepared plan. I explained to the victim that Medjet had basically refused to come, that Global Rescue was ready with a few moments notice, but that it may cost him more than $100,000 since he didn't have their coverage. He gulped and said to call them. I sat up with the victim for most of the night. He had a few assistants with him from his corporation who were instructed to inform me of any changes while I slept nearby for a couple of hours. I had discussed with Global Rescue that, if he deteriorated, they could not wait until morning as planned and would have to come in the dark, despite the difficulties of evacuation at 9000 feet. Signal fires would need to be lit because it would be difficult to locate us. It would be a dangerous extraction in those circumstances. Though he appeared relatively stable, I still did not know if the victim had internal hemorrhage from splenic or liver injuries, a closed head injury, or non-displaced fractures. Believe me, it was a welcome sight to see the large green Peruvian military helicopter which looked like a large grasshopper appear over the horizon early in the morning.

The rest of the expedition left for the canyon, and I remained with the patient. The alcalde (mayor) of the area remained with me along with two Peruvian guides. We got the patient situated in the helicopter and he waved goodbye with his bandaged hand and a smile.

I then proceeded down the mountain with the guides and the alcalde. It was very steep, and they elected to put a guide in front and one behind me with a rope between them on my outside in case I fell. They got a big laugh when I remarked that it looked like they were bringing a prisoner to jail.

Global Rescue made a large, beautiful poster about this experience for marketing. The narrative of the rescue was set against a backdrop of the explorer team marching single file along the narrow trail among the breathtaking Andes mountains.

This situation highlights one of the important points I make about travel protection. You need to understand what coverage you are paying for. The contract I reviewed claimed in big letters at the top MEDICAL EVACUATION but in the fine print text it stated only medical transportation. This could mean transport by ox cart to the next village. In this case, the victim had the financial means to pay for his evacuation, but this cost could be a huge burden for a lot of travelers. Later, as I gave presentations about expedition medicine and used this situation as a teaching point, the Medjet lawyer had the audacity to send a nasty letter asking me to cease and desist from disparaging the company. I promptly made that letter my next slide in the presentation, demonstrating how some of these companies persisted in not doing the right thing, going after the doctor instead of fixing their inadequacies.

A year or so later, I noted that Medjet had altered its policies to explain its covert coverage more clearly. However, I still recommend another company.

I have become good friends with the victim who's a very successful Texas oilman, very humble and quiet about his circumstances. He flew me on his jet to his "hacienda" in southern Texas where he is revered by his employees and the town of Laredo, Texas. We still talk on a regular basis, and he says he prays for me every night for which I am indeed grateful.

Another patient on this trip had severe back pain such that he could not walk anymore. Suspecting muscular back spasms, I treated him with muscle relaxants which effected a miraculous cure for him. He is an accomplished photographer in New York and every time I see him, he tells everyone around him that I saved his life in the Andes. It was not that dramatic, but I understand the gratitude for significant pain relief.

Piotr held an annual kayaking event in West Virginia for his key clients and has taken me twice to kayak. The Gauley River is arguably considered the most difficult Class V rapids to traverse in the eastern U. S. These are made even more turbulent when the government opens the dams twice a year. Of course, that is when Piotr would go. Some of these rapids dropped several feet and kayakers had to hang on for dear life and then paddle frantically to steer. Piotr had a photographer positioned such that when the drop occurred, he would get great photos of us in the throes of this frightening experience. I was in the raft with Terry Garcia, executive VP for National Geographic and John Rasmus, editor of National Geographic Adventure magazine and I remember slamming into Terry rather hard. For years I had to listen to him tell me I was to blame for the demise of his golf game because his swing was interfered with due to injuries. I did slam into him rather hard, so it was within the realm of possibility. He got a lot of mileage out of that story for sure.

Over the years, Piotr would call me when he would go to remote areas, particularly in South America, while he was exploring with National Geographic for the source of the Amazon. These are high altitude regions where consideration needs to be given for the use of prophylactic medications to prevent high altitude sickness. There are various presentations of this syndrome with the most dangerous being high altitude cerebral edema (HACE) and high-altitude pulmonary edema (HAPE). Both conditions involve swelling and retention of fluid in critical organs like the brain and lungs and can kill the victim if not reversed. The most used medication is acetazolamide (known as Diamox) and then steroid use in an emergency. In addition to carrying these meds, it is advisable to bring a broad-spectrum antibiotic to deal with pulmonary infections. Climbers must acclimate to the altitude over a few days to avoid these problems. There are side effects to consider such as dehydration because Diamox is a diuretic, meaning that one urinates more while using it. Coupled with the dehydration that occurs at higher levels, constant replacement of fluids is important.

Piotr contacted me urgently when there was an impending problem with Aleksander Doba, a renowned kayaker who was the 2015 National Geographic Adventurer of the Year. He was attempting his third solo kayak crossing of the Atlantic and they had lost contact with him near Bermuda. I was unable to join him immediately and communicated with Piotr when he went to Bermuda to look for Doba in a boat. As they were circling the area, they spotted the kayak drifting near Bermuda. Fearing the worst, they approached the covered kayak shouting his name.

Finally, he stuck his head out of the top but explained he could not come out yet, he had no clothes on. Over the course of the trip from Europe to Bermuda, his waterlogged clothes had started to fall apart so he had removed them, and he feared there were females on the approaching boat. They finally were able to persuade him to get out and ascertained he was physically fit but embarrassed.

Piotr called one day and asked me to help him with a potentially dire situation. A couple of Polish explorers were deep in the Amazon and one of them rappelling to look at petroglyphs (old carved figures on rocks) had placed his arm on a ledge right in front of a large snake that bit him on the shoulder. The guide identified it as a fer-de-lance, a highly venomous pit viper. Piotr asked if I could help get the explorer evacuated. It was now ten hours after he had been bitten. They were trying to get him evacuated with assistance from the Polish ambassador and the Columbian military, but the military wanted $50,000. Since the man was still alive, I suspected that he may have sustained a dry bite, meaning little or no venom was injected but we could not be certain, and he would need wound care and a tetanus shot.

While Piotr was dealing with the politics, I contacted medical colleagues in Colombia who confirmed that the man should go to the military hospital in Bogota, the best source for the fer-de-lance antivenin. My colleague arranged for the victim to be transported there. The Colombian military decided to perform this helicopter rescue as a training exercise and for good will. Because this area is quite dangerous due to narcotic traffickers, the military sent two choppers, one for the rescue and a second one to circle and protect the rescuing helicopter. The choppers searched for three hours trying to find the explorers and just when they were ready to give up, they located them deep in the jungle on a river (as they had been instructed). The basket retrieval to the hovering helicopter was precarious but accomplished; the victim was evaluated by the military physicians who came to the same conclusion, he had a dry bite. Still, he was very lucky.

A photo sent to me showed a three-inch gap between fangs in his shoulder. He had been bitten by a very big snake. One humorous sidelight to this was that as the choppers hovered over the small boat, a man suddenly dove overboard, swam to shore, and dashed into the jungle. He surfaced three days later in another town. We were told he was wanted by the military and bailed out to avoid them recognizing him.

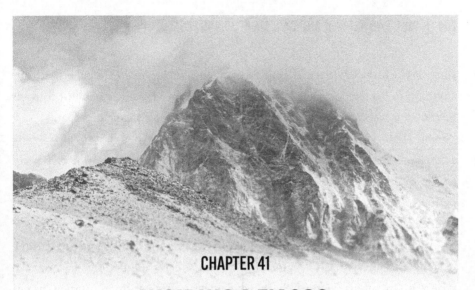

CHAPTER 41

AVOIDING A FIASCO: PANAMANIAN PETRGLYPHS

S ometimes it was fortuitous to avoid an expedition. The Peruvian trip was precarious because of the terrain but a Central American opportunity turned out to be dangerous for other reasons. A local Explorers Club chapter member claimed that he had evidence for an unknown new pre-Columbian civilization in Panama on the border right above the country Colombia in an area known as the Darien Gap. That area is a rugged, jungle covered area that still is not controlled by the national military. The Darien Gap is the only area where the Pan American highway is incomplete as it stretches all the way from Alaska to Tierra del Fuego.

His phantasmagorical story was that on a birdwatching trip in that area he met an indigenous native of the Embera tribe, one of the groups which populated that remote region. He invited the native Daniel back to Washington and helped him get connected to the Georgetown University linguistics school who began to compile the first dictionary of the Embera language. He asked Daniel if there was anything to explore in that area and the native said he could take him to ruins unknown to western world science. They went back to Panama and Daniel took him on a half-day trip back into the jungle on a pirogue. They came to an opening at the confluence of two medium-sized rivers where there were a lot of pottery shards and evidence of an old city. There were also large examples of prominent petroglyphs or stone carvings. The explorer wanted to mount an expedition to return and evaluate the ruins further.

In the meantime, I was asked to speak in Panama and had a chance to visit the Panama Canal, a fantastic engineering marvel still surrounded by an American zone. On my off afternoon I chartered a small motorboat to go up the Chagres River and visit the Embera village which interfaced with tourists. It was oppressively hot and humid but the tattooed and painted indigenous people were fascinating and served us lunch on a palm leaf. On the way back, I learned a valuable lesson about the jungle and how you can become hypothermic in a steaming jungle, something I had been quite skeptical about previously. A rain squall popped up on our return trip and soaked us. Despite light rain gear, I shivered violently after the storm all the way back to our car. I promptly got hot chocolate in the rainforest roadside café. While I got a taste of the terrain and climate, I certainly did not expect a freezing experience.

Back in Washington, I saw photographic evidence of the petroglyphs and the Darien Gap site littered with pottery. I offered to help him because he would certainly at least need medical advice. He had been in sporadic contact with Dr. Carlos Fitzgerald, purportedly a prominent Panamanian anthropologist. There was little progress, however, as I watched for three years, I asked the chapter member if he wanted assistance in organizing the expedition. There was a prominent Panamanian medical oncologist in research at GWU also affiliated with several major Texas hospitals. When I was given permission to be more involved, I contacted Dr. Adan Rios for his thoughts. His close friend was the current vice president of Panama, and he connected us. We decided to do a site visit to Panama to prepare for a larger expedition.

The small team I put together included Tim Friend, the science writer from USA Today and an independent movie producer who had worked with National

Geographic. When we arrived in Panama, I arranged to meet with the vice president and his staff to discuss the expedition. The vice president asked why we had stalled, and my explorer friend replied that Dr. Carlos Fitzgerald was now not responding to him. The VP turned to his assistant and said, "Get Dr. Fitzgerald on the phone." Fitzgerald promptly answered. The VP then explained that he expected his cooperation. The stagnation ended.

We then were to meet with the native Daniel. We waited two hours and he finally appeared roaring drunk. It quickly became apparent that he was a middleman trying to weasel his way to a fee for introducing us to the actual Embera tribe. We were disappointed and I began to get the feeling this expedition was a bad idea.

This intuition was confirmed when I returned to Washington and consulted with my security friends. The consensus was clear and not ambiguous, do not go. Scott Harrison told me that his sources said there are two mountain chains in the isthmus of Panama where the Darien Gap is located. Between the ranges and on either side were rivers, which were the only means of transportation. The area is a hotbed of narco-terrorists, and they would most certainly know we were there. The narcos would decide if it was worth their while to kidnap us and hold us for ransom. My friend had been very lucky in the past because he sneaked in by himself and got out quickly. That likely would not be our fate on the proposed longer trip with more people to attract attention.

I pulled the plug on this South American expedition but continued to look for more suitable opportunities.

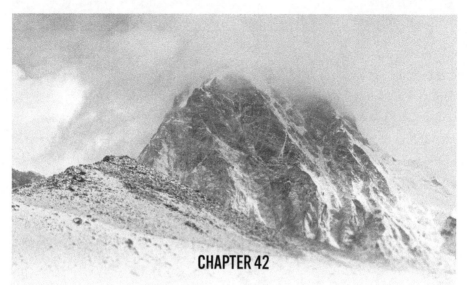

CHAPTER 42

BACK TO MONGOLIA: A NEW CAMEL SPECIES

Afaster returning from the Andes, a good friend of mine from the Club called me and said she was unable to go on an amazing expedition and would I like to take her place to Mongolia again! The location was 800 miles into the Gobi Desert, one of the most formidably hostile environments on earth. We were to join John Hare, OBE, and Fellow of the Royal Geographic Society, at the breeding site he had created for the third species of camel on earth. John had spent more than two decades in discovery and education for the world about this animal, *Camelus ferus*, the wild camel. Most people are aware of the one-humped Dromedary camels that tourists ride in Egypt, and many are aware of Bactrian camels, a distinct species with two humps. This very rare third species is quite unknown to the public.

I knew John Hare from The Explorers Club; he is the quintessential British explorer right out of central casting, with an impeccable vocabulary and manners. John was a biologist who had been with a Russian expedition to the Taklamakan Desert which straddles the Chinese and Mongolian borders in a desolate area that China had used to test nuclear bombs (43 of them) because they thought nothing lived there. The wild camel had just been formally identified six months before our trip as an entirely distinct species through DNA testing at the breeding site. The ancestors of this two-humped camel diverged from the ancestral camel line 700,000 years before the common ancestor of today's Bactrian and Dromedary camels. There are less than 1000 wild camels alive separated in three distinct populations under severe environmental stress.

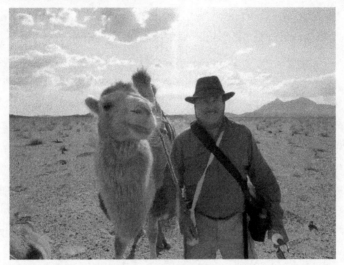

Riding camels deep in the Gobi Desert in search of the newly-described third species of camel, the wild Bactrian Camelus ferus.

This was indeed intriguing, and I contacted another explorer, Colonel Don Morley (ret) USAF engineer whom I had taken on the Titanic expedition. Our studies of light transmission at 2.5 miles down in the ocean proved the premise of blue light transmission of information in that difficult environment. Don is another road warrior who always brought different gadgets useful in remote areas. He enthusiastically agreed.

My brother-in-law, Tim Dennis, had been hounding me to take him on an expedition for some time. He founded a steel company and isn't an explorer. He needed to know that we would be driving for three straight days across some of the most hostile geography on earth, would have neither showers nor bathroom facilities for about ten days, and would have to ride camels for a couple of days.

This would not be a picnic, but it would be very interesting. Although he was a little anxious about it, he agreed immediately.

We met up with a tour guide in the Mongolian capitol Ulan Bataar, home to half of the population in this vast country. There were evident changes in the city, compared to my first visit, likely from the influx of foreign capital interested in the extensive mineral resources in Mongolia. We hopped in our Range Rover and left for the desert in the middle of summer when it was hot in the day, but the temperature plummeted to just above freezing at night. Each night we pitched our small tents in the desert by the very sparse roadside and cooked our meals. We did not encounter another soul on the road. The British tour guide James was delighted to turn over some of the cooking duties to Tim who was a good cook.

Tim's culinary skills were especially welcome later in the trip when we were running out of food supplies on a cold, rainy day with miserable horizontal rain while we were on camel back. John Hare had joined us on a two-day camel ride to a special spiritual place known as Mother Mountain. We decided to take the day off after this bone-jarring last four days on the Range Rover and camels. We got to an area with the hut-like gers (also known as yurts) and Tim scrounged up vegetables and made the very best tomato soup that I have ever had. He made a huge pot, and we ate it with relish for both lunch and dinner. It really warmed us up as well.

We were in the middle of nowhere, literally, and woke up the next day to a commotion. It seems it was a holiday in Mongolia and a group of teachers had come out to this spiritual area. Mongolians like to drink, so they had started early and now about noon, they were curious about our group of obvious foreigners. A few of them staggered over. They spoke no English, but our Mongolian driver figured out they were teachers. They kept coming over, perhaps expecting that we had gifts for them. My brother-in-law Tim was not amused that I told them he had all the money. We did give the teachers a few things and they left the next day.

Back at the breeding facility, a few of the wild camels in a large enclosure were to be evaluated for breeding possibilities. I was able to go on foot to within 30 yards of one of them which was quite a thrill to see such an endangered species up close. What spurred the interest in these camels was the fact that they would come out of the wilderness to mate with domestic Bactrians during mating season.

Originally thought to be escapees from the Silk Road caravans of earlier centuries, John Hare was one of the first to question that premise which led to this project and the discovery of an entirely new species.

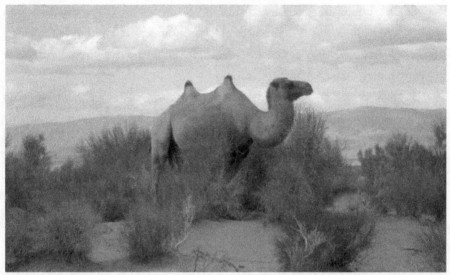

The Bactrian wild camel *Camelus ferus*. There are less than one thousand of these very ancient camels in the wild.

We had a great evening around the campfire where John said we each had to sing a song from our cultures. Our off-tune singing was abetted by John who had us generously sample the alcohol fermented from mare's milk. This process involves different individuals (Mongolians) taking a big mouthful of the new milk, swishing it around, and then spitting it into a container which then ferments over a few weeks to create a quite powerful alcoholic drink. Only God and a microbiologist knows what microbes are in there. I did reassure our group that I had broad spectrum antibiotics that covered just about everything in case somebody got sick. This was not my favorite pastime, but we got through it.

After a few days to observe the breeding station, it was time for us to go. We departed on the barely visible road which was now obscured even more by the heavy rains which had returned. Contrary to its reputation as a desert, it rained in biblical proportions for a few days, and we were running out of food. It was with growing concern that I watched our excellent Mongolian driver surveying the "road" for alternative pathways. It was time to go. By the time we got to a hotel a few days later in Ulan Bataar, we would have killed for a shower and restaurant meal. Those who have lived in austere circumstances understand how great that shower feels.

After a day or so, we departed Mongolia. I had told Tim that I never went straight back home after such an expedition because we needed to ease back into real life over a couple of days. Tim had reluctantly agreed, and we headed to Hong Kong to catch up with my close friend Scott Harrison who now lived there and in Manila while running his security company.

Tim was amazed at Hong Kong, one of my favorite cities. We spent four days there decompressing from Mongolia. Tim now wholeheartedly agrees with my philosophy to ease back into our culture, and we were now ready to re-engage in our busy lives.

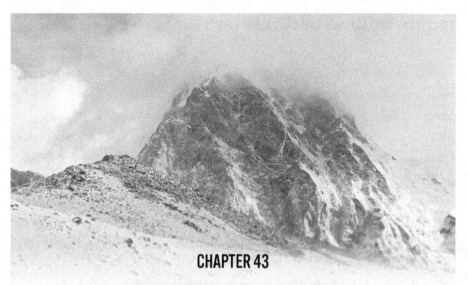

CHAPTER 43

ANCIENT FOOTPRINTS

R ight before I began my stint at Triple Canopy as chief medical officer, I had another unique exploration opportunity. I reviewed student grants for TEC and ran across one that intrigued me. Once again it involved paleoanthropology. A grad student in geology at Appalachian State University applied for a grant to join her professor in northeast Tanzania to evaluate a brand-new finding of suspected early human footprints.

Lake Natron is located in northern Tanzania in Africa's Great Rift Valley, close to the border. This shallow lake is less than ten feet deep, and the water level varies significantly between rainy and dry seasons.

As water evaporates during the dry season, salinity levels increase promoting growth of salt-loving microorganisms. These salt-loving organisms use plants to produce energy. Red pigment in the cyanobacteria produces the deep reds of the open water and the orange hues of the shallows of the lake. These colors are characteristic of lakes with very high rates of growth. In addition, the salt crust on the surface of the lake is often colored red or pink by the cyanobacteria.

Lake Natron is the only breeding area for the 2.5 million endangered Lesser Flamingoes that live in the valley. As salinity and cyanobacteria increase, the flamingoes flock along saline lakes in the region to feed on these blue-green algae with red pigments. However, Lake Natron is the only breeding location for Lesser Flamingoes because its environment is a barrier against predators trying to reach their nests. The temperatures in the mud can reach 50 degrees C (120 degrees F), and depending on rainfall, the alkalinity can reach a similar level to ammonia. Amazingly, an endemic species of fish, the alkaline tilapia, also thrives at the periphery of the hot spring inlets in these ordinarily inhospitable waters.

> We had an ornithologist who explained that flamingoes originated in East Africa in this area. Flamingoes were imported to North Africa and the Romans then imported them to raise them for their tongues as a delicacy. Spain imported flamingoes and then the US imported flamingoes from Spain to Florida, so our flamingoes originated in Africa. The fiery swarms of nearly 10,000 flamingoes leaving at sunset to nest at Ngorongoro crater are strikingly beautiful.

The area around Lake Natron turns out to be exactly like the lake my son Tim and I visited a couple of years ago where we saw soda ash being mined at Lake Magadi in southern Kenya near the Tanzanian border.

Because of threats to the salinity balance from projects in Natron watersheds, such as a planned power plant, and proposed development of a soda ash plant at Lake Natron, Tanzania named the Lake Natron Basin to be preserved on July 4, 2001. Destruction of this breeding site would be devastating to the Lesser Flamingo population.

The Ngare Sero Tented Camp was developed in 2004 around a recently discovered spring on private land leased from the Maasai in the sparsely inhabited northern border of Tanzania. This small comfortable camp is an attractive location for birders to view the flamingoes of Lake Natron and other bird species and animals attracted to the spring waters. In 2006, a Maasai herder tending the small herd of camels at the camp came across footprints in the volcanic ash about a ten-minute drive from the camp. Preliminary indications suggested that these prints were old enough to generate scientific interest. With permission from the

Maasai, a small group was headed to the area under Dr. Cindy Liutkus-Pierce, the geology professor whose grad student was applying for a grant to join.

I contacted Dr. Liutkus-Pierce, introduced myself, and gave her my credentials. She was close to the Smithsonian paleoanthropologists who urged her to take me on the trip. This was the first scientific evaluation of the prints in August 2009, and we excavated and mapped the visible prints and uncovered several more.

Known fossil hominin footprint sites are extremely rare and range widely in age and location from about 350,000 years in Europe to the most famous track dated to 3.6 million years in Tanzania. These dates are constantly pushed back by new discoveries. Footprints provide important information about the biomechanics and behavior of our bipedal ancestors while clues about paleoenvironments, paleoclimate, and preservation mechanisms can be determined from studies of the geology surrounding footprint sites.

Game abounded at the fossil site, including many wildebeest, zebra, giraffe, jackal, and some oryx. I heard hyenas near the tent but did not see any. There were no large predators because the Maasai keep them out to protect their cattle. Lots of birds cavorted especially around the camp which surrounded a clear spring that created a small lake.

The camp was a 10-minute drive from the footprint site. The whole place is in the shadow of a large volcano, Ol Doinyo Lengai, one of two active volcanoes in Africa. The peculiar landscape had all kinds of large volcanic rocks that had been spewed out by the volcano.

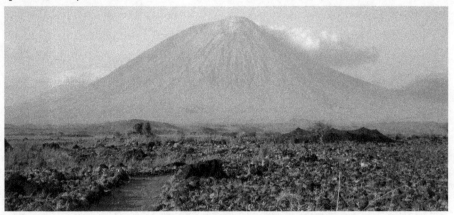

Ancient Homo sapiens footprints found in the shadow of active volcano Ol Doinyo Lengai in rural Tanzania.

The footprint site was in the shadow of this active volcano, in the middle of a windswept area intermittently inundated by floodwaters. The impressions in the volcanic ash are very well preserved with frequent exquisite detail; volcanic ash mixed with water makes cement. Rain often accompanies volcanic eruptions so maybe that was the source of water. Right next to the ash was a lava flow so it may very well be that there are more prints under the old flow. The lava had large rocks that had been shot out of the volcano and made a still visible splash as they landed. The rocks (called pyroclasts) were a little bit elongated because they stretched and cooled as they were shot out of the volcano creating a very distinct geological picture.

There were twenty-four prints evident when we arrived, heading in a direction away from the volcano. There were only six of us, including two Tanzanians from the Department of Antiquities, so the excavation and documentation kept us quite busy. We uncovered more than thirty more prints for a total of fifty-eight. I found nine myself, many of them in excellent shape.

We had to shovel first gently, then brush, then chip the layer of ancient sediment above the ash gently to find prints. It was thrilling to uncover a curve that turned out to be a toe or heel. There were at least three individuals, probably two men and a woman. The woman's track was 20 meters long. One man had about a size 14 foot and a stride 6 inches longer than mine so he must have been at least 6 foot 4 inches or so, very unusual because the humans of that era were thought to be shorter, with an average around 5 feet 6 inches or so. The other man (presumably) seems to have been close to 6 feet tall with about a size 10 foot. Just like me. We measured each print, the stride lengths, and charted and photographed them. The tracks appeared to go right under a sand dune. This was confirmed a few years later when a major expedition with footprint experts documented a village with over 500 prints some from small children.

This has become a world heritage site dating back to about 19,000 years before the common era (BCE). Many of these Homo sapiens prints had all the toes clearly visible. Current fossil and genetic evidence point to the origin of modern humans in Africa about 200,000 years ago. These footprints are being studied in detail to reconstruct gait, speed, and tentative body weight and height. Chemical composition of the ash will be compared to that of the regional volcanoes to determine the origin of the footprint-bearing ash. The findings will lead to multiple publications.

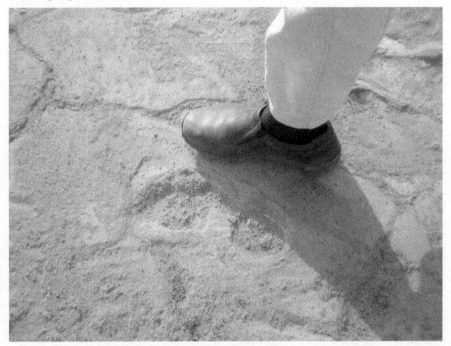

Over 500 footprints over 19,000-years-old have been uncovered at this world heritage site including whole families on the move.

After six days and delightful visits from the Maasai elders in the surrounding villages who promised to guard the prints, we left for Arusha. On the way, we stopped at Laetoli, the site of the oldest and most famous human prints, dating from 3.6 million years left by very early ancestors of humans, the australopithecines (like Lucy). These print tracks are much shorter in length and now have been covered up since 1997 to protect them. However, the dirt used for cover had seeds in it and acacia trees sprung up causing root damage to the site. The resulting controversy is how to protect the prints we found and there is much speculation about how to do that. The president of Tanzania has declared that they cannot be covered so the public cannot see them. It is an unanswered question. I hope to participate in that next step.

We also had a great side trip to Olduvai Gorge, the most famous site of early human fossils starting with the Leakeys in the 1930s and 40s. Louis Leakey's son

Richard, a very famous paleoanthropologist who recently died, had continued the work for almost fifty years. It was he who first suggested to Rick Potts to excavate the highly productive site at Olorgesailie in the Kenyan Rift Valley area.

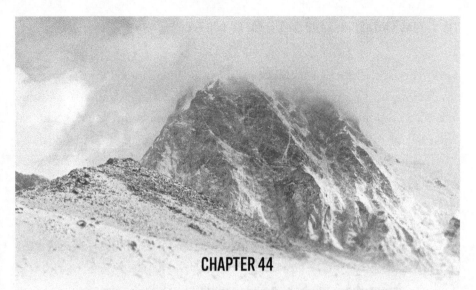

CHAPTER 44

THE WORLD EXPLORER PROGRAM
AND THE EXPLORATION MERIT BADGE

onsulting work and expeditions continued, and I donated my time to another passion, Eagle Scouts. I had been asked in 2012 to join the National Eagle Scout Association (NESA) committee which functioned as their board of directors. My old friend from The Explorers Club, noted speleologist Bill Steele, was the director. This was quite an honor. I was being dragged back into the tent, figuratively, many years after leaving scouting. After a meeting shortly after my acceptance in 2013, Bill asked me to investigate sending Eagle Scouts to Antarctica. In 1926, the BSA sent an Eagle with Admiral Byrd on his first reconnoiter of the South Pole. The Eagle, Paul Siple, became very excited about meteorological research and chose that for his career, later inventing the wind chill factor.

Over the course of the next eighty-five years, BSA had been able to send an Eagle or two sporadically back to Antarctica and now NESA, the organization under BSA which dealt with Eagle Scouts, wanted to continue this on a more

217

consistent basis. The major problem was that now international treaties governed any activity in Antarctica. That means that American organizations or private individuals desiring to do Antarctica research had to apply through the National Science Foundation, which was a difficult process, particularly for individuals.

I turned to Bill and NESA president Glenn Adams and said, "Why are we only going to Antarctica? I know many explorers going to very interesting places and we should go all over the world to mountains, jungles, the ocean, and other venues."

A lightbulb went on as they saw the expanded possibilities. I received the approval to proceed, and we created the NESA World Explorer Program with seed funding. I tapped into my large network and created a pilot program where we sent an Eagle with a science teacher to the Amazon Tiputini Biodiversity Station (TBS) in eastern Ecuador, located deep in some the best Amazonian rainforest. It was imperative for me to evaluate safety, transportation, ability to evacuate in case of an adverse event, local facilities, and other issues before I could look parents in the eye and assure them it was safe to send their sons deep into the jungle or other austere environments.

I contacted fellow explorer and friend, Colonel Chris Macedonia, an MD whom I had brought to the Titanic salvage expedition and sent to Everest. Chris had a background in expedition medicine and was project manager at the Defense Advanced Research Project Agency where he was exposed to the latest classified technology under development. Chris was a resourceful guy to travel with to remote places and readily agreed. We arrived in Quito, a beautiful city high up in the Andes, and contacted the University de San Francisco Quito. The 6.5 square kilometers of TBS is jointly administered by Universidad San Francisco de Quito in collaboration with Boston University. Established in 1995, it provides a field research venue in rainforest abutting the Tiputini River which has been restricted from hunting of large mammals in agreement with the indigenous people. It is not easily reached because of its remote location. Field scientists and students perform research on a wide variety of scientific and environmental interests. The university controlled and ran the Tiputini Biodiversity Station.

Ecuador is a small gem of a country with picturesque Quito nestled in the Andes bisecting the unique Galapagos Islands and some of the most biodiverse rainforest in the world. We flew early the next day by small commercial plane for two hours to Coca, a regional city close to the Amazon rainforest. There we were brought to an outrigger motorized canoe and proceeded down the Napo River for another three hours, then departed on a bus for a rural three-hour ride, only to board another motorized canoe on the serpentine Napo.

We passed through a small security entrance at the last boat launching site and came across a small group heading back from the site. We had not seen anyone else on this trail and these were obviously Americans, so I hailed them, and we introduced ourselves. They were from Culver, Indiana, a small town well known for the military academy there. I told them I had gone to college just north of there, in South Bend, and the lead guy, an Ecuadoran, whirled around and asked," Did you go to Notre Dame?" It turned out we graduated the same year from ND. We told him about the Eagle Scout site visit, and he stated that he was the provost of University de San Francisco Quito in charge of these programs with former high school classmates and friends. He invited me to the university when we returned. I could not believe my luck, Dr. Carlos Montufar was the exact person I needed to talk to for permission and I ran into him in the middle of the rainforest.

His parting comment to me as he turned to go was that he also oversaw their Galapagos program. The Galapagos Science Center is a hotbed of marine biology research. This was incredible news for now I would have a second spectacular program for Eagle Scouts. The time spent in the biodiversity camp was magical. The biologists and our guide were very knowledgeable, pointing out insects and animals we may not have noted, including the trail of fire ants running frantically up my pant leg. I learned I had some new dance moves.

There were at least ten different camouflaged large insects like walking sticks, like the one that looked like a partially eaten leaf, brown and green, that if had not moved you would never notice. We had the highly endangered pink freshwater dolphins cavorting around us while on the river. Stunningly brilliant blue morpho butterflies flitted around. Many diverse colorful and exotic tropical birds including the large and wild looking hoatzin hopped among the hugely diverse panoply of plant life. Incredible plant diversity included walking palms and huge fig trees (ficus), a lot larger than your domestic house plants, and the majestic ceiba trees, some of them 100 feet tall with trunk circumferences up to 30 feet. Peccary scat was all over the place, but we did not want to run into a pack of these wild pigs. Jaguar prints were also seen periodically, a reminder that these beautiful big cats were plentiful in the forest. Jaguar scat with teeth in it testified that at least part of the jaguar diet consisted of the peccary wild pork. We did not see a jaguar, unfortunately, but they were there. One of the biologists told me a melanotic (black) jaguar popped its head up about 50 feet from where he was working recently and stared at him. Although Tiputini was home to the largest population of ocelots in the world, we did not see any. We did see the large rodent capybara on several occasions and saw its natural predator, the anaconda, fully stuffed (probably with capybara) snoozing on the riverbank.

A night walk with the guide revealed a different set of rainforest characters. We spotted colorful or camouflaged snakes though fortunately none were venomous. Different large spiders monitored webs in confined spaces awaiting prey. We skirted a large centipede or millipede, but we did not stop to count the legs which likely had tiny hairs that can produce a very painful response. We also saw diurnal poison dart frogs, startlingly bright among the foliage.

A whole other world existed in the forest canopy. Tiputini had an incredible series of rope suspension bridges 50 feet up in the treetops. These were built by another close Explorers Club friend Dr. Meg Lowman, also known as Canopy Meg, famous for her research in this unique environment. Up in the trees, howler monkeys and other primate species pirouetted from limb to limb right in front of us. A whole different ecosystem of insects inhabited these environs. Tarantulas hung out very close to our treetop walkways. Various birds eyed us as they hopped by looking for insect meals. Back in the camp for breakfast we were joined by a huge spider one morning, a huntsman species, like my old spider friends in Africa.

Returning in awe back to Quito, Dr. Montufar invited me to join him and his friends for lunch. This was at the Culinary Institute of Ecuador, housed at the university, and we had the fantastic head chef give us a cooking lesson in Peruvian cuisine, considered by many to be the finest in all Latin America. Seated across from me were the two key scientists from the university who ran field operations at Tiputini. Dr. Montufar had placed us together to work out the details for the

Eagle Scout activities. We got along famously and set up the program which we implemented when I returned home.

Returning home, we now had two great programs for Eagles in exploration. I began to add to the program destinations. Our only real limitation was the funding I would receive from NESA and the BSA to expand.

After the initiation of the World Explorer Program and due to my involvement with the NESA committee, I was asked to be a speaker at the BSA National Jamboree in 2015. This national event attracted 40,000 scouts and roughly 300,000 of the public. This was a very nice honor, and I would share the program with a few other prominent speakers. One of them was Dr. Lee Berger, a well-known paleoanthropologist who had the great fortune to discover two new early human species within the last few years. These discoveries adorned the front pages of newspapers and covers of prestigious magazines around the world.

Lee and I had a great time speaking to the scouts and we both wondered why the Boy Scouts did not have an Exploration merit badge. We queried the national leaders the next day and they responded that it was a great idea and that we should submit a proposal. So, Lee and I sat in a smoky bar in West Virginia and outlined on a cocktail napkin the tentative requirements to earn the Exploration merit badge. The draft outline was presented to an enthusiastic senior leadership. I was asked to write the formal proposal and the booklet accompanying the merit badge that went to all scouts seeking the merit badge. We now could reach nearly 2 million scouts with exposure to exploration.

Here is an excerpt from the beginning of the Exploration merit badge booklet that outlines the concept of exploration and the requirements needed to earn the badge:

"Have you ever wondered about your surroundings and wanted to learn more about them? Have you thought about the natural world and its interactions? Have you wanted to know why a machine works or an insect flies or what triggers some animals to hibernate? Have you been intrigued about the invisible world around us…. bacteria, molecules, viruses, wind currents, tides, x-rays? Have you taken a walk in the woods just to see what is over the next ridge? Then you are interested in exploration!

These are natural urges that are inherent in humans. While not all of us want to jump in a kayak and traverse the Amazon, the truth is that no other mammal moves around like us according to evolutionary anthropologists. Several scientists are exploring the human genome to see if there is a genetic basis for this urge in our species. You see, this search in itself is exploration, and it is being done in a laboratory.

Anthropologists, neuroscientists, and other researchers have repeatedly tied a variant of a gene to certain characteristics of explorers. This gene controls a chemical messenger within our brains known as dopamine which is important for learning and reward. The variant of the dopamine gene has now been shown in many studies to be strongly related to curiosity and restlessness. About 20 percent of the human population has this variant gene which makes them more likely to explore new places, ideas, food, and other behaviors. These people tend to seek movement, change, and adventure. Animal studies of this gene variant show similar behavior of increasing interest in movement and new things.

In humans, this genetic variant has also been strongly linked to human migration and that peoples with nomadic lifestyles have a higher incidence of it in their populations. While this variant has sometimes been called the "explorer gene", the urge and ability to explore is likely more complicated. But this variant gene may be a stimulus in our large capacity human brain to explore. Certainly there are people without this variant who have interest in exploration but this may be an added influence in some.

Exploration has been defined as the search for discovery of information or resources. In scientific research, exploration is one of the three basic principles that guide research along with description and explanation. So discovery, description, and explanation make up the essence of research…..and exploration (discovery) is a key component.

Exploration is the engine that drives innovation whether it is in science, economics, or commerce. We really need exploration to drive medical discoveries to help mankind, to seek alternatives for being more energy efficient, to protect our planet's resources, to better understand the impact of our oceans and atmosphere, and to look at extraterrestrial environments."

The Boy Scout merit badge committee asked for my opinion regarding the logo for the Exploration merit badge. They sent me a series of activities such as mountain climbing, scuba diving, hiking, and similar activities. Most were too generic, but one stood out to me. It was a depiction of a classic fedora hat on top of binoculars, clearly an Indiana Jones facsimile. The model for Indiana Jones was Dr. Roy Chapman Andrews who in 1922 discovered dinosaur eggs in Mongolia while wearing such a hat and pearl-handled pistols to fend off Chinese bandits. He was my first hero and a member of The Explorers Club so to me this was perfect. The only thing missing was the whip. When I brought that up the committee was aghast stating that the whip would send the wrong message of violence and subjugation. I retorted that everyone knew the whip, it was part of the Indiana Jones persona. Shortly after that, I was invited to give a seminar on how to become an explorer for a very large Boy Scout meeting of the Order of the Arrow, a semi-elite subset of scouts. In my presentations to more than 1,000 Scouts, I asked for their opinion about the logo. In both sessions, numerous scouts asked about the missing whip. I smiled as I thanked them and took those comments back to the merit badge committee. The boy scouts had spoken, and the iconic whip was added.

It would be a fantastic opportunity for Eagles in the NESA World Explorer program to go to South Africa and participate in paleoanthropology research with Lee and his field team. I detoured when I was speaking in South Africa to visit Lee and he took me to both discovery sites, a huge thrill to see early hominin fossils of *Australopithecus sideba* still in the ground. These are tentatively dated to around 1.9 million years old. We also went to the discovery site of *Homo naledi*, found by recreational cavers, in the Rising Star cave system. This proved to be a treasure trove of hominin fossils of at least 21 individuals, amounting to over 2000 specimens, estimated to be 236,000 to 350,000 years old. Their place in the evolutionary chain before dying out appears to be a mixture of terrestrial and arboreal environments.

We were able to send Eagle Scouts for a few years to these sites located in a game reserve near Johannesburg. When we were not looking at amazing fossils we were on the lookout for game. The drives through the reserve got us up close to giraffe, elephant, zebra, rhino, kudu, and many other antelope species.

We did find a leopard den on foot, which had me nervously looking over my shoulder. Once back in Johannesburg, we spent time in the lab with world class scientists from various countries, evaluating the fossils and learning about their unique characteristics.

The World Explorer program that I developed with strong support from NESA leaders Bill Steele, Glenn Adams, and Frank Tsuru became a focal point for BSA and NESA marketing. About three percent of Boy Scouts become Eagles. Eagles had to be finished with scouting and interested in sciences but not already started in a career. They had to be at least eighteen-years- years old, therefore adults in the eyes of the law, and accomplished in service to their community. Most years we had around 300 Eagle Scout applicants for the fourteen spots available. These were some of the very best Eagles, true stars in waiting for all walks of life though most in this program were likely to be involved with science.

In addition to the Amazon biology and the Galapagos for marine biology, we sent Eagles to South Africa but also for paleontology to excavate dinosaurs at the Montana site of the largest dinosaur found in North America. We deployed them to Yellowstone with the NASA Astrobiology program addressing the question of whether life exists beyond Earth, and how humans can detect it. They conducted photochemical experiments of thermophilic biofilms in hot springs to simulate reactions that took place on planetary surfaces. Another program sent Eagles to the Michigan upper peninsula to band bald eagles with noted ornithologist Bill Bowerman and to study effects of pollution and pesticides. Eagles also participated in speleology in the huge Mammoth Cave system where every year they published data to extend the length of the longest cave system in North America. Two Eagles traveled in separate years above the Arctic Circle to work on narwhals with Smithsonian expert Dr. Martin Nweeia. One of them also contributed to the book accompanying the permanent exhibit on narwhals in the National Museum of Natural History. He went on to change his college major to curatorial science and is now a museum curator. This is a perfect example of our program having a lasting effect on a young man's career. One year we conducted a jungle survival school with Special Forces where scouts foraged for edible greens and built rafts to cross a river. Now that young women have been admitted to the scouts, we will have stellar candidates from this constituency. Lastly, twenty of these Eagles have now joined The Explorers Club and have a full expedition under their belt, a welcome addition to the Club rolls. I am very proud of this achievement.

> During all this, I was named a Distinguished Eagle Scout (DESA) which requires national prominence in your field or career. Only 0.1 percent (1 in 1000) of Eagle Scouts attain this designation. Since 3 percent of scouts attain Eagle, that translates to 3 in 100, 000 scouts receiving the DESA award. My award came as a surprise announcement at a Boy Scout national meeting where I was speaking in front of over 600 attendees. The standing ovation was very gratifying.

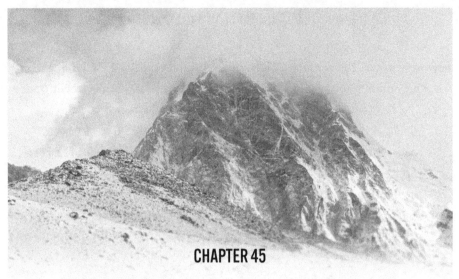

CHAPTER 45

THAI SOCCER TEAM CAVE RESCUE

A most singular opportunity arose in October 2018 when I was a speaker at an international medical conference in Sydney, Australia. In July 2018 worldwide news emerged about the Thai youth soccer team trapped in a flooding cave system that were rescued from certain death by a daring group of cave divers. Cave diving is another form of insanity in my mind. The doctor who had orchestrated the rescue and made the decisions about how to sedate these youths was an Explorers Club Fellow and Australian chapter member.

I contacted Dr. Richard (Harry) Harris and introduced myself as an associate editor of The Explorers Journal. I wanted to both do my regular column on expedition medicine on cave diving and perhaps do a larger article on this rescue. I was very surprised when Harry said, "Mike I know exactly who you are, I have both of your books on expedition medicine on my desktop at all times." What a compliment from this explorer!

I flew the two and a half hours to Adelaide where he is the medical officer for the search and rescue team for the state of South Australia. Harry is an anesthesiologist in addition to cave diver who has published about underwater cave rescues. Cave diving medical emergencies have a high mortality. We compared notes about evacuation and management of field emergencies and then he enthralled me with his firsthand account of the Thai soccer team cave rescue. The interview for The Explorers Journal told the amazing story well depicted in the movie *Thirteen Hours*.

The movie differed from reality in that Harry made the medical decision about whether and how to sedate the young men. This type of rescue had never been attempted and he told me he expected to lose about half of the boys. They lost none. The burden of this decision makes this rescue even more noteworthy. Harry, however, sustained a personal loss because his father died while he was on the rescue, a very sad epilogue indeed.

But Harry is MY hero, what he did was amazing. I still get goosebumps thinking about what he accomplished. This excerpt is how I ended that article: "One could easily paraphrase a famous quote from Antarctic explorer Sir Raymond Priestley about Ernest Shackleton after his famous rescue of his men: 'For scientific discovery, give me Scott; for speed and efficiency of travel, give me Amundsen; but when disaster strikes and all hope is gone, get down on your knees and pray for Shackleton.' It seems very appropriate to substitute Harris for Shackleton when it comes to cave diving disasters."

I stand by that statement in my admiration for what Dr. Harry Harris did. His rescue efforts epitomize expedition medicine.

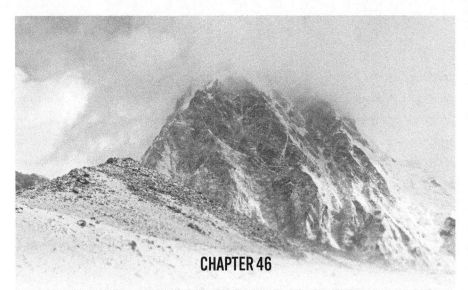

CHAPTER 46

INFECTIOUS DISEASE BIOSURVEILLANCE AND COVID

A major disruptor of normal life appeared at the end of 2019 with the emergence of the SARS CoV-2 respiratory coronavirus. I was the Chief Medical Advisor for Crisis Response for Accenture from 2012 to 2019; Accenture is a 600,000 plus employee business support corporation with a high concentration of employees in India and southeast Asia. These areas are hotbeds of disease activity and concern for infectious disease experts because of high population density and intersection with potential animal hosts such as those in the live markets of China. Because of my background in both security and tropical medicine, Accenture wanted me to help monitor bad diseases throughout the world. There was justifiable concern about one of the deadly flus gaining the ability to easily infect humans, which would be a pandemic disaster. There were a few bad actors that gave us the most concern, like bird flu, swine flu, MERS (Middle East Respiratory Syndrome) coronavirus, and

SARS, a coronavirus luckily contained in China before escape. Then there were the unknowns.

We had been monitoring various outbreaks of disease such as Ebola which has periodically erupted in west and central Africa. This disease has a case fatality rate of 50 percent but fortunately this primitive organism has very fastidious requirements which helps contain its spread. We are all easily connected these days through international airline flights so that something can readily escape and be transmitted around the world quickly. I attended National Security Council meetings regarding Ebola where a policy was crafted to address future outbreaks and to stockpile key supplies. Had this been implemented, we would have had supplies that could have been deployed for the subsequent Covid pandemic. In fact, there is another outbreak of Ebola in Uganda as this is being written in 2023.

I presented the latest updates on infectious disease problems with the potential to affect employees or interrupt business to the global security team at Accenture three times a year. In addition, they wanted my input about their pilot bio-surveillance program established in Manila, Philippines. This program used a rapid genetic sequencing application to identify the organism in patients with respiratory symptoms appearing in the emergency room of the most advanced hospital in Manila, St. Luke's Medical Center. This program was also used to evaluate patients with suspected dengue fever and the results showed that at least 10 percent of them had a similar though less dangerous disease called Chikungunya with the same symptoms of fever, joint aches, and muscle aches. They had not seen any evidence for flu viruses.

Accenture sent another medical employee on this site visit to inspect the machinery and its use and any clinical results. The chairman of St. Luke's board of directors and chief medical officer was my old professor from University of the East, Joven Cuanang, a brilliant Harvard-trained neurologist.

Dr. Cuanang was legendary at University of the East (and I suspect wherever he went) because he would introduce his class on the first day by simultaneously drawing with both hands mirror images of both cerebral hemispheres with brainstem. Dr. Cuanang and I quickly caught up with each other on what we had be doing and why I was at his hospital.

He strongly suggested that I go to the infectious disease center of the Philippines because another University of the East grad was the director. We had a very productive meeting in addition to quick access to the sequencing machine and physician in charge.

Of course, I took my security colleague to visit the Hobbit House while in Manila.

Back in the States in November 2019, I saw a small article that reported a few patients with an unknown respiratory viral disease who had died. I could not find any further information about this. I contacted Accenture and DXC, a similar business information corporation for whom I consulted. I told them that we needed to monitor this combination of events. Companies began to explore contingencies for business interruption and employee health in case this became a real problem. Unfortunately, it did. It was the very beginning of the coronavirus pandemic.

As events unfolded over the next two years, the global security team met every two weeks for updates as the world shut down. RNA viruses like coronavirus mutate very rapidly since they have single-stranded genetic material. The expression of that mutation is much easier to manifest than in a double-stranded (DNA) virus where mutations in both mirror-imaged genes were usually required for manifestation of the change. I warned them that this virus would mutate, and that viral evolution usually followed a pattern of increased infectivity but less lethality. That activity may render a vaccine obsolete. At that time, long covid began to appear. I and others advised the company that this disease would be with us for quite a while with this mutation pattern and that long term care would likely be an issue. This information was used by senior management to formulate corporate policy that is still an ongoing issue.

Meanwhile, we continue to monitor other diseases. Both seasonal flu and another respiratory virus, Respiratory Syncytial Virus (RSV), are now raging through populations no longer sequestered but with no immunity. Some nasty, highly resistant fungal infections are surging particularly among intensive care units and other pockets of immunocompromised patients and threaten to overflow into the general population. Malaria still kills about 3 million people a year and has now developed resistance to the latest medication.

We continue to be in an arms race between small organisms and medical therapy.

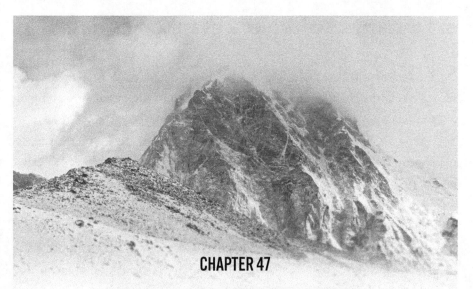

CHAPTER 47

WHAT IS ON THE HORIZON?
THE NEXT EXPEDITION

I am often asked what my favorite expedition is, and my wise-guy response usually is "the next one." Anticipation of the next adventure or intriguing medical issue has defined much of my life. I certainly could not have anticipated some of my life's great adventures either in exploration or the medical field. My age and health may limit future activities. Maybe now I can finally dismiss that looming Everest shadow that crops up periodically.

A domestic adventure with exploration might be just the ticket and so I have become involved in one of the enduring mysteries in the bird world. The story of the Ivory-billed Woodpecker (IBW), our largest woodpecker, is complex and controversial. The last widely accepted sighting of this species in continental North America was 1944, documented with photos. Despite continued sporadic but poorly documented reports of sightings by fishermen and hunters, the U.S. Fish and Wildlife Service recently proposed declaring the species extinct.

However, ornithologists at Cornell University in 2005 presented audio recordings of the IBW's very distinctive nasal call and pattern of drumming on trees in Arkansas from the Mississippi riverine bottomland forests, the classic preferred IBW habitat. They only had a brief, blurry video clip that is suggestive but not conclusive of the IBW. In 2022, the US National Aviary in Pittsburgh published an elegant manuscript on ten years of research in Arkansas trying to document the existence of the IBW. The data accumulated including calls, evidence of bark stripping unique to this bird, and video that looked very much like an IBW and its typical flight pattern strongly supported the theory of continued IBW existence. They now have an intriguing video that looks like an IBW.

I had discussed this with a close friend for many years, world renowned Mayo Clinic medical oncologist Dr. Oliver Sartor who is an amateur and quite knowledgeable bird watcher. Oliver and I have worked on several projects together over the years since we first met at the National Cancer Institute when he was on staff during my fellowship. Oliver hails from Louisiana and is a member of a small group with homes in a 7000-acre private tract of land in Mississippi just above the Louisiana border across the river adjacent to the Arkansas area of interest. Their seven miles of Mississippi River waterfront is a stunning vista, and you feel like Huck Finn with your feet up on the porch rail on the river at his hunting lodge. He has a perfect base of operations to search for this elusive bird.

In 2022, we conducted a site visit of this alternate source of habitat with ornithologist Peggy Shrum from the U.S. National Aviary. The habitat matches that of the IBW, and we found evidence of their unique holes drilled into dead trees for nesting. There was bark stripping, also unique to these woodpeckers in the quest for their favorite grubs. Pileated woodpeckers, another large but ubiquitous species, likely made the transition to ants as their primary food source some time ago as civilization continues to encroach on the habitat. The IBW still seeks the grubs that are even more scarce because of the changing landscape. The grubs persist in these woodlands.

The site visit is a prelude to a larger expedition after the US National Aviary ornithologists gather definitive evidence this spring of the IBW's continued existence from a prospective nesting area. That will be front page news. I look forward to participating in some capacity with the larger expedition. After all, they may very well need a physician in the vicinity, there are some huge venomous snakes in that lowland swampy area....

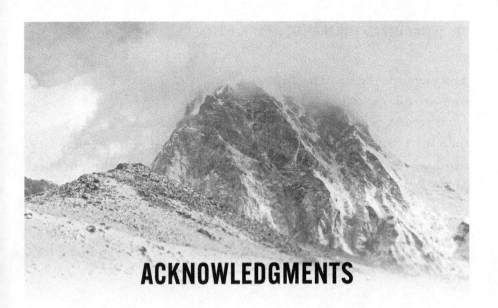

ACKNOWLEDGMENTS

Writing a book is a daunting task, and an author often needs assistance traversing the many components of bringing the story to a finished product. This is certainly true for me, and I offer very heartfelt acknowledgments to the following. You have all been editors in one respect or another, and your contributions have been essential. Any errors in the text are truly mine.

Firstly, to my formal editor and content confidant, Debby Englander, without whose help this would still be in a formative stage. She provided editorial guidance and direction for the stories and for which publishers might be interested. I owe her a great deal of thanks.

Likewise, a hearty thanks to Elizabeth Brim for her editorial oversight and advice. She has been very reassuring in our approach to publication.

Mary B. Riddle and Ian Iraola provided essential and much-needed direction for a social media platform and marketing strategy. Without them, I would still be floundering in these arenas. Furthermore, their unflagging positive support was critical to the completion of this book.

The team at Morgan James Publishing, headed by David Hancock, included Isaiah Taylor, Gayle West and her team, and others who weighed in on content and organization. They also provided editorial oversight for which I am eternally grateful.

Of course, much like Sir Arthur Conan Doyle's Sherlockian Baker Street Irregulars, I had my host of informal experts who helped with context and corrected impressions. Rachel, Susanna, and Timothy Manyak headed that bunch with assistance from friends.

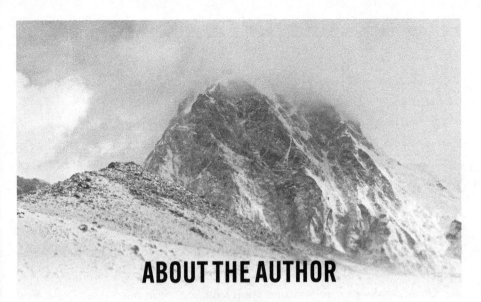

ABOUT THE AUTHOR

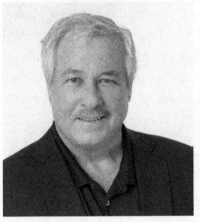

Dr. Michael J. Manyak (1951 - 2024) was an explorer, author, urologist, and corporate medical executive. He served as the Chief Medical Advisor for Crisis Response for Fortune 500 companies and for the Greater Washington (DC) Board of Trade.

A Distinguished Eagle Scout, an honor bestowed upon only 0.1% of Eagles, Dr. Manyak actively shaped future generations of explorers. As Vice President for the National Eagle Scout Association (NESA), he directed the NESA World Explorer Program and spearheaded the development of the Exploration Merit Badge. His dedication to the field is further evidenced by his authorship of over

250 professional abstracts, book chapters, and refereed journal articles, alongside 11 patents.

Dr. Manyak's recently published book, *Lizard Bites & Street Riots: Travel Emergencies and Your Health, Safety & Security*, addresses health, safety, and security for travel emergencies. This insightful guide was a finalist for both the USA Best Books Awards and the International Book Awards for travel guides and essays in 2016.

A National Fellow of The Explorers Club and a former Board of Directors member for 10 years, Dr. Manyak actively contributed to the organization's prestigious journal, *The Explorers Journal*, through his column on Expedition Medicine.

Dr. Manyak's passion for exploration led him to lead or serve as the medical director of diverse expeditions around the globe. These included ventures to the Titanic, the Central African jungle, Antarctica, the Peruvian Andes, Mongolia and the Gobi Desert, Tanzania and Kenya for paleoanthropology, and the Amazon rainforest. Throughout his remarkable career, he collaborated with esteemed organizations like NASA, National Geographic, and the Smithsonian.

A free ebook edition is available with the purchase of this book.

To claim your free ebook edition:

1. Visit MorganJamesBOGO.com
2. Sign your name CLEARLY in the space
3. Complete the form and submit a photo of the entire copyright page
4. You or your friend can download the ebook to your preferred device

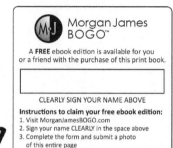

Morgan James
BOGO™

A **FREE** ebook edition is available for you
or a friend with the purchase of this print book.

CLEARLY SIGN YOUR NAME ABOVE

Instructions to claim your free ebook edition:
1. Visit MorganJamesBOGO.com
2. Sign your name CLEARLY in the space above
3. Complete the form and submit a photo of this entire page
4. You or your friend can download the ebook to your preferred device

Print & Digital Together Forever.

Snap a photo

Free ebook

Read anywhere

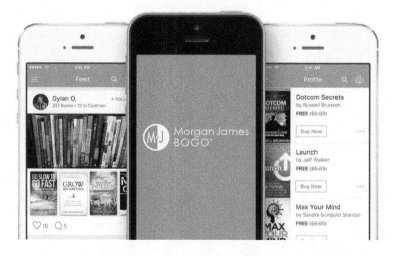

www.ingramcontent.com/pod-product-compliance
Lightning Source LLC
Jackson TN
JSHW081500070125
76711JS00004B/45

* 9 7 8 1 6 3 6 9 8 3 9 3 6 *